Palliative Care for South Asians, Hindus, Muslims and Sikhs

i

Other titles available in the Palliative Care series:

Fundamental Aspects of Palliative Care Nursing by Robert Becker and Richard Gamlin

Palliative Care for the Child with Malignant Disease edited by the West Midlands Paediatric Macmillan Team

Palliative Care for People with Learning Disabilities edited by Sue Read

Palliative Care for the Primary Care Team by Eileen Palmer and John Howarth

Why is it so Difficult to Die? by Brian Nyatanga

Palliative Care for South Asians, Hindus, Muslims and Sikhs

edited by
Rashid Gatrad, Aziz Sheikh, Erica Brown

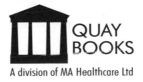

QUAY
BOOKS
A division of MA Healthcare Ltd

Quay Books Division, MA Healthcare Ltd, St Jude's Church, Dulwich Road, London SE24 0PB

British Library Cataloguing-in-Publication Data
A catalogue record is available for this book

Printed in Malta by Gutenberg Press, Gudja Road, Tarxien PLA19, Malta

To 7816   WT
600
PAL

iv

CONTENTS

List of contributors   vii

Foreword by Sir Liam Donaldson   ix

Introduction   xi

Acknowledgements   xvii

Section One: The Basics

1   National guidance on palliative care   3
     John Linnane

2   Developing culturally competent services in palliative care:
     management perspectives   11
     Paula McGee, Mark RD Johnson

Section Two: A Question Of Faith

     Introductory comment — The language of religious symbolism:
     rendering visible the invisible   29
     Sabina Gatrad, Rashid Gatrad

3   The Muslim grand narrative   33
     Sabina Gatrad, Rashid Gatrad, Aziz Sheikh

4   Palliative care for Muslims   41
     Rashid Gatrad, Aziz Sheikh

5   The Hindu grand narrative   57
     Shirley Firth

6   Palliative care for Hindus   69
     Rashid Gatrad, Pam P Choudhury, Erica Brown, Aziz Sheikh

7   The Sikh grand narrative   83
     Jagbir Jhutti-Johal, Sukhvinder S Johal

8   Palliative care for Sikhs   95
    Rashid Gatrad, Hardev Notta, Sukhmeet Singh Panesar,
    Erica Brown, Aziz Sheikh

Section Three: Delivering Care

9   Improving communication and access to palliative care
    through the arts   103
    Dipti P Thakker, Christina Faull

10 South-Asian mothers with a life-limited child
    at Acorns Children's Hospices   117
    Erica Brown

11 The transition from paediatric palliative care to adult services   131
    Erica Brown, Karen White

12 Reflections of a Macmillan nurse   147
    Glenys Mitchell

13 Multi-faith chaplaincy   155
    Andy SJ Lie

14 South-Asian perspectives on bereavement   167
    Shirley Firth

Glossary   183

Appendix — Agencies working with South-Asian communities   191
    Sally Killian

Index   195

LIST OF CONTRIBUTORS

Erica Brown is Head of Research and Development, Acorns Children's Hospices, Birmingham, UK

Pamela P Choudhury is Consultant in Palliative Medicine, St Giles Hospice, Lichfield, Staffordshire, UK

Sir Liam Donaldson is Chief Medical Officer, Department of Health

Shirley Firth, formerly Lecturer in World Religions, Death and Dying (Open University), Death in the Asian Tradition (MA), universities of Reading and Winchester, UK, is a freelance lecturer and writer

Christina Faull is Consultant in Palliative Medicine, University Hospitals of Leicester and the Leicestershire and Rutland Hospice, UK

Rashid Gatrad OBE is Professor of Paediatrics, University of Kentucky, USA; Consultant in Paediatrics, Manor Hospital, Walsall, UK; and Senior Lecturer, University of Birmingham, UK

Sabina Gatrad is in her final year of a BA degree in philosophy

Jagbir Jhutti-Johal is Lecturer, Department of Theology, University of Birmingham, UK

Sukhvinder Singh Johal is Senior Research Fellow, Multidisciplinary Assessment of Technology Centre for Healthcare (MATCH), University of Nottingham, UK

Mark RD Johnson is Professor and Director, Mary Seacole Research Centre, De Montfort University, Leicester, and the NHS Specialist Library in Ethnicity and Health, UK

Sally Killian is Manager of Cancer Information and Support Services, Walsall Teaching Primary Care Trust, UK

Andy SJ Lie has served on the Church of England's Inter Faith Consultative Group since 1996 and is currently Chief Executive, BECON, based in north-east England

John Linnane is Deputy Director of Public Health Medicine, Walsall Teaching Primary Care Trust, UK; and Chairman, Black Country Palliative Care Network, UK

Paula McGee is Professor, Faculty of Health, University of Central England, UK

Glenys Mitchell is Clinical Nurse Specialist in Palliative Care

Hardev Notta is Asian Liaison Officer, Interpreter for Acorns Children's Hospice, UK

Sukhmeet Singh Panesar is a medical student, Imperial College, University of London, UK

Aziz Sheikh is Professor of Primary Care Research & Development, Primary Palliative Care Group, Division of Community Health Sciences: GP Section, University of Edinburgh, UK; and Chairman, Research and Documentation Committee, Muslim Council of Britain

Dipti P Thakker is a member of the Oncology Department, Cancer Centre, University Hospital, Birmingham, UK

Karen White is Adolescent Team Leader, Acorns Children's Hospice, UK

FOREWORD

Enabling people to have choice over where they live and die is an incredibly important part of patient care. People who have come to the end of curative treatment should be treated with dignity and respect so that care at the end of their lives can meet their individual needs. Providing high-quality end-of-life care to all who need it should be a real marker of success for the NHS. However, because of an historical failure to appreciate the subtleties of different cultures' attitudes to death, people from minority groups have not always received this care. By focusing on the physical and psychological affects of death, and assuming that all people need or want the same model of care, we fail to meet the needs of ethnic-minority groups at this vital point in their lives. Any contribution to reducing this unacceptable inequality in palliative care is welcome.

This book provides anyone working in palliative and supportive care with an important tool for working with people from South-Asian communities. Its multidisciplinary approach, taking expertise from medical, nursing and community professionals, sets out a framework for ensuring that the diverse needs of this group are appreciated. The principles and practice of palliative care are funded on the basis of responding not only to physical and psychological factors, but also to the spiritual, religious and emotional aspects of death, which are just as important to patients and their carers. This book places an understanding of different religious attitudes to death at the core of palliative care, developing a broader understanding of how we treat patients at the end of their lives. It also makes an important case for making palliative care available to non-cancer patients, and, given that ethnic-minority communities typically have higher death rates from diseases other than cancer, this is also important in reducing inequality at the end of life.

The NHS is committed to improving the standards of palliative and supportive care and to reducing inequality. The End of Life Initiative, launched in 2004, provided £12 million pounds over three years to improve the care of terminal patients. This initiative is supporting the introduction of the *Gold Standards Framework* and the *Liverpool Care Pathway for the Dying*, as well as the *Preferred Place of Care* tool. These tools will allow greater choice for all patients, and will enable palliative care to be applied to a broader range of conditions. It is important that these approaches do not ignore cultural and religious diversity. It is vital that the lessons of this book are acted on by professionals and policy-makers.

Sir Liam Donaldson
Chief Medical Officer
Department of Health
December 2005

INTRODUCTION

The opportunity to die with dignity is recognised by health professionals the world over as one of the most fundamental of all human rights. However, what is often forgotten is that notions of a 'good death' vary considerably between cultures (and individuals within a culture), raising the risk of misunderstanding, pain and anguish for all those who are left behind (Helman, 1998).

But this need not be the case. Even in ethnically and religiously diverse societies, such as ours in modern Britain, receiving high-quality care at the end of life is possible and may, we hope, soon be a liklihood for all (Department of Health [DoH], 2000; Hill and Penso, 1995). Realising this aspiration will require fundamental changes on at least three fronts:

- tackling institutional discrimination in the provision of palliative care;
- progress in incorporating transcultural medicine into medical and nursing curricula; and
- a greater willingness on the part of healthcare providers to embrace diversity and, in so doing, develop a richer appreciation of the challenges facing people from minority communities in achieving a good end (Hendry, 1999).

The introduction of palliative care into health care is a relatively recent phenomenon, and even now these services are mainly focused on the needs of elderly people dying from cancer. However, migrant communities in Britain are typically younger and have proportionately higher death rates from diseases not related to cancer, such as diabetes and cardiovascular diseases (Firth, 2001). Other factors may contribute to the difficulties in accessing appropriate terminal care. These include the belief among some that hospices, with their Christian roots, cater only for white Christian communities and that hospitals have 'unreasonable' restrictions on visiting times and numbers of visitors for dying patients.(Gatrad and Sheikh, 2002).

No effective national provisions are in place for the training of health professionals in transcultural medicine, and few professionals will therefore have had any real opportunity to learn about death rites in different cultures. For example, why is it that a middle-aged Muslim daughter insists on maintaining a day-and-night hospital vigil of her dying mother? (Sheikh and Gatrad, 2000). Or why is it that a Sikh man with end-stage renal failure persists in describing 'pain in his heart' when he really means he is upset? (Gatrad and Sheikh, 2002). And why is it that a terminally ill Hindu patient wishes to die as close to the floor as possible? (Gatrad et al, 2003). The importance of these and other rites of passage need to be understood by caregivers.

So how do we move forward? The continuing evolution of palliative-care services is crucial to ensuring that minority ethnic and faith communities have access to high-quality terminal care. Important developments have, however, taken place in community palliative care, with the widespread introduction of Macmillan nurses and children's hospices. Priorities must now include services that embrace people with a much broader range of terminal conditions; these include end-stage renal, lung and cardiac failure, which are important causes of death within minority ethnic communities, particularly South Asians (NICE, 2003).

We need proactive strategies to recruit staff from a diversity of backgrounds (Alexender, 2003). Our experiences show that multifaith hospital 'chaplains' and minority ethnic outreach workers represent a particularly valuable resource in helping to overcome language barriers. In addition, they can help develop services and promote partnerships with local communities (Gatrad *et al*, 2003).

Health professionals are increasingly encouraged to focus on the idea of a good death. However, definitions have not included a religious perspective, but have tended to emphasise physical and psychological dimensions. These often include control of symptoms and help with resolving 'unfinished business'. Issues to do with faith — a subject so important to so many people during their last days — need to be incorporated into mainstream professional training. An estimated sixty-five medical schools in the USA now offer modules on spirituality and health, and these examples of good practice need to be emulated in Britain (Koenig *et al*, 2001).

But even the best training cannot cover all aspects of care nor deal with many ways in which values and norms interact and adapt before finally being enacted in the hospital, surgery or home. To help push such an agenda forward, we have, however, a relatively untapped potential for penetrating insights into how to shape the future for the provision of palliative care: the doctors, nurses and allied health professionals who, with their broad range of ethnic, religious and cultural backgrounds, represent a most valuable learning resource.

Our aim in this book is to attempt to provide an answer to the crucial yet elusive question of how best to improve the end-of-life care available to South Asians and their carers. In seeking to help move discussions forward beyond the rhetoric and consider how best to translate good intentions into actual improved care, we draw on contributors, in this book, who represent a broad range of academic disciplines, including epidemiology, social sciences, humanities, the arts, theology and diversity studies. Our clinical and allied health professional contributors, who have equally diverse backgrounds, share their experiences and expertise of working in a range of healthcare settings, incorporating primary-, secondary- and hospice-based care. The religious and spiritual perspectives of our authors are also varied; we are particularly fortunate to have contributions from those who live, work and breathe within the three religious faiths that are a focus of study in this book, thereby allowing, perhaps for the first time, a truly 'insider's perspective' of being heard.

Linnane opens with an overview of a spate of recent national policy directives, which have triggered an expansion of traditional approaches, and encourage the development of novel approaches, to delivering supportive and palliative care. McGee and Johnson in *Chapter 2* provide an in-depth discussion of the management considerations that are essential to translating these polices and legal developments into action in the context of end-of-life care. Then, to set the scene for the six following chapters (*Chapters 3–8*) on religious grand narratives and end-of-life considerations for each of the three faith groups under study, Gatrad and Gatrad provide a brief but necessary *Introductory comment* on the language of religious symbolism in the context of the lived faith experiences of British South Asians. Together, these represent the first two sections of the book, looking at trends in the development of palliative care and cultural competence, and exploring the implications of these issues, in a generic sense, to those who live and die within faith-based world-views.

The third section focuses on the practicalities of delivering care to those with life-limiting illnesses and begins with a fascinating account by Thakker and Faull (*Chapter 9*) of their highly innovative (and successful) attempts to improve understanding of, and access to, palliative care for South Asians through three interlinked arts-based projects, one of which involved working with young people through the medium of rap music. This theme of working with younger people is continued in the following two chapters (*Chapters 10 and 11*) by Brown, which are based primarily on her wealth of experience with young South Asians that she accrued working at the widely respected Acorns Children's Hospice, Birmingham, UK.

In *Chapter 12*, using an in-depth personal case-study approach, Mitchell movingly reflects on the dangers of stereotyping and the ease with which, despite the best of intentions, this can be done. This is followed by a passionately argued chapter on the question of 'multi-faith chaplaincy' (*Chapter 13*), where Lie fundamentally challenges the widely held notion that progress in equality of provision of chaplaincy care to minority faith communities is being made: Lie's central theme is that progress will only really be achieved when power-structures within hospital chaplaincy units change. The final chapter allows Firth to develop further some of the issues raised in her previous chapter on the Hindu grand narrative (*Chapter 5*), and broaden this discussion by offering a conceptual basis for framing the variety of bereavement responses manifested by Muslims, Hindus and Sikhs. The work concludes with a glossary serving as an *aide memoir* of key terms that are used in the text, but which are not indigenous to the English language, and an appendix of organisations and services with a particular interest in the provision of end-of-life care.

The net result of this work is, we hope, a text that will inform, challenge, provoke and, at the same time, move readers to reflect on how, together, we can facilitate improved delivery of care to our South-Asian communities.

We have in this work consciously focused on exploring the needs and care of three core sections of the South-Asian community: Muslims, Hindus and Sikhs. This approach raises some potentially important theoretical limitations that warrant consideration. One might, for example, very reasonably ask why we have focused on only these three faith groups when there are other important religious communities from South Asia, such as Buddhists or Christians, who have now also made their homes in Britain. There are, in addition, increasing numbers of South Asians who may only subscribe nominally to a religion, or have no religious affiliation at all. One might also ask — to what extent do the discussions in relation to, say, Islam or Hinduism, which are arguably more global religions than Sikhism, also hold true in relation to Arab or European Muslims or East-African Hindus? To a certain extent, this last question is addressed in an earlier work in relation to Muslim care in which two of us (AS and ARG) were involved (Sheikh and Gatrad, 2000), and by a pending work on the care needs of Hindu patients (Thakrar and Sheikh: forthcoming).

Our decision to focus on these three religious traditions has been motivated by a combination of theoretical and pragmatic considerations. Despite the decline in religious affiliation in many parts of the world, our experiences — which are reinforced by findings from the 2001 UK census (available at http:/www.statistics.gov.uk) and the 2004 Home Office Citizenship survey (O'Beirne, 2004) — suggest that, for the majority of British South Asians, religion continues to play an important role in defining their identity, particularly at crucial turning-points of life, such as death and bereavement. These three religious faiths represent by far the largest groupings both in the Indian Sub-continent and here in Britain; also, and perhaps more importantly, these are communities about which we and our co-authors can, on the basis of our experiences, claim a degree of expertise, whereas the same would not necessarily have been true had we chosen to cast our net wider.

We acknowledge that this work represents but a first step in what still remains largely uncharted territory. Nonetheless, our hope is that the impact of this (admittedly confined) work will set in motion a broader ripple in the ongoing discussions of diversity and health inequalities, extending beyond these groups (South-Asian Muslims, Hindus and Sikhs), locality (Britain) and perhaps even (end-of-life) phase under study.

Understanding each others' narratives of what constitutes a good life and good death offers us the possibility of improving the quality of care we deliver. The added benefit is that this helps us as individuals make better sense of questions that we will all encounter at some stage in our lives: how do I want to live, and die?

Rashid Gatrad
Aziz Sheikh
Erica Brown
December 2005

References

Alexander Z (2003) The Department of Health study of black, Asian and ethnic minority issues. www.doh.gov.uk/race_equality/ziggistudy.pdf (accessed 8 Jul 2003)

Department of Health (DoH) (2000) *The NHS Plan*. Stationery Office, London

Firth S (2001) *Wider Horizons*. National Council for Hospice and Specialist Palliative Care Services 21, London

Gatrad AR, Sheikh A (2002) Palliative care for Muslims and issues before death. *Int J Pall Nurs* **8**: 526–31

Gatrad AR, Choudhury PP, Brown E, Sheikh A (2003) Palliative care for Hindus. *Int J Pall Nurs* **9**: 442–8

Gatrad AR, Rehana Sadiq, Sheikh A (2003) Multifaith chaplaincy. *Lancet* **362**: 748

Helman C (1998) *Culture, Health and Illness*. Butterworth-Heinemann, Oxford

Hendry J (1999) *An Introduction to Social Anthropology: Other People's Worlds*. Macmillan, London

Hill D, Penso D (1995) *Opening Doors: Improving Access to Hospice and Specialist Palliative Care Services by Members of Black and Ethnic Minority Communities*. National Council for Hospice and Specialist Palliative Care Services, London

Koenig HG, McCullough ME, Larson DB (2001) *Handbook of Religion and Health*. Oxford University Press, Oxford

NICE Guidance No 5 — published Oct 2003: *Chronic Heart Failure — Clinical Guideline for Management in Primary and Secondary Care*

O'Beirne M (2004) *Religion in England and Wales: Findings from the Home Office Citizenship Survey*: p. 9

Sheikh A, Gatrad AR (2000) Death and bereavement: an exploration and a meditation. In: Sheikh A, Gatrad AR (eds) *Caring for Muslim Patients*. Radcliffe, Oxford

Sheikh A, Gatrad AR (eds) (2000) *Caring for Muslim Patients*. Radcliffe, Oxford

Thakrar D, Sheikh A (eds) *Caring for Hindu Patients*. Radcliffe, Oxford (forthcoming)

UK Census (2001) Available online at http:/www.statistics.gov.uk (Last accessed May 2005)

ACKNOWLEDGEMENTS

Andy SJ Lie wishes to thank Dr Dermot Killingley for his advice on an ethically delicate matter and Christina Faull for her support and encouragement.

John Linnane wishes to thank Helena James and Gill Yardley.

Rashid Gatrad gives his sincere thanks to Josephine Jones for her help and patience during the preparation of this book.

Shirley Firth wishes to thank *The Lancet*.

Sukhmeet Panesar says, 'All that I am and ever will be, I owe to my mother.'

The editors wish to thank patients and their carers for allowing them to use their narratives. To protect their anonymity, all names and ages of patients have been changed. Note Greenhough, etc. The Introduction (p. *xi*) in this book is an cxpanded and adapted version of an editorial published in the *British Medical Journal*: Gatrad AR, Brown E, Sheikh A (2003) Palliative care needs of minorities. *BMJ* **327**: 176–7. The editors also thank Hardev Notta.

Christina Faull and Dipti P Thakker are indebted to those taking part in the SAPCA and all those who allowed them to use their artwork in this book.

For our parents, with love.
RG, EB, AS

Civilisation is judged by the treatment of its minorities.
Mohandas 'Mahatma' Gandhi (1869–1948)

Section One:
The Basics

CHAPTER 1

National guidance on palliative care

John Linnane

May the Lord support us all the day long,
till the shades lengthen and the evening comes,
and the busy world is hushed, and the fever of
life is over, and our work is done!
  John Henry Newman

This chapter outlines some recent innovations in palliative care service policy and provision. It is recognised that the availability and quality of care available for oncology patients and those with other life-limiting diseases may be variable across the UK (Edmonds, 2004). The need to extend the palliative-care approach to other groups of patients has been highlighted by the publication of guidelines for professionals caring for patients with heart failure (National Institute for Clinical Excellence [NICE], 2003) and chronic obstructive pulmonary disease (COPD) (NICE, 2004). The implementation of the new contract for GPs in April 2004 (GMS2), with its emphasis on improving primary care management of a range of chronic diseases, is another significant development (Gomes and Higginson, 2004).

Recent legislation has also highlighted the importance of service provision in palliative care. In 1999, the Department of Health (DoH) launched the *National Carers Strategy* legislation, which emphasised the importance of service provision that enabled families caring for children and adults with complex health needs to maintain an acceptable lifestyle, including paid employment if they wished. Additionally, the physical and mental health of carers and the opportunities they have to integrate into their local community was highlighted.

The following year, a commitment towards palliative care was outlined in *The NHS Cancer Plan* (2000) and endorsed by Prime Minister Tony Blair

---

Panel 1.1: Policy developments since 1996

- *The NHS Cancer Plan (2000) and the establishment of palliative care networks.*
- *The Gold Standards Framework.*
- Targeted investment in palliative care services (2003).
- *Building on the Best: Choice, Responsiveness and Equity in the New NHS (2003).*
- The New General Medical Services (GP) Contract (2003).
- Long-term Conditions and Expert Patient Programme (2003).
- *NICE Guideline on Supportive and Palliative Care (2004).*
- *National Service Framework for Long-term Neurological Conditions (2005).*

---

in his commitment to review palliative-care services. The result has been the publication of a number of important documents, including some that have had specific implications for patients from black and ethnic-minority groups. The NICE *Guidance on Cancer Services* (2004) is of particular relevance.

Additional NHS resources have also been provided for palliative care. In 2002/3, the Government provided a non-recurring allocation of £10 million for palliative-care services. A number of areas were identified to receive this ring-fenced revenue, which was primarily allocated in recognition of the contribution of the voluntary sector to the provision of palliative care. This resulted in most of the resources being transferred to adult hospices.

An additional £50 million allocation was made available for the next three years, fulfilling an electoral promise by the Government to pump prime further development of palliative-care services across England and Wales. Several criteria for allocation of funds were identified. These included the need to address gaps in service provision at a local level, ensuring that the requirements of the then draft NICE guidance on supportive and palliative care would be adequately addressed. There was an expectation that, at the end of the three-year period, the resource requirements would be mainstreamed.

A range of policy developments either directly targeted at improving palliative-care services or pertaining to related service areas has been issued over recent years and is outlined below (*Panel 1.1*).

NICE guidelines for improving supportive and palliative care for adults with cancer

In March 2004, NICE published detailed guidance for the NHS on supportive and palliative care. While initially directed at services for people with cancer, there remains an expectation that the recommendations of the guidance will be extended to include support for patients with other life-limiting illnesses such as diseases prevalent amongst South-Asian communities relating to diabetes, cardiovascular disease and renal failure. Although the guidance acknowledged a lack of evidence for many of the key issues identified, the framework sets out a number of service models. These models were designed to ensure that patients, their families and carers receive support and care that will help them cope with their illness and its treatment at all stages, including the end of life.

The NICE (2004) guidance includes twenty key recommendations for the development of supportive and palliative care. A summary of some of the key issues addressed is presented in *Panel 1.2*.

Panel 1.2: Key developments in supportive and palliative care

- coordination of care
- service user involvement
- face-to-face communication
- information
- psychological support
- social support
- spiritual support
- general palliative care, including care of dying patients
- specialist palliative care
- rehabilitation
- complementary therapy
- care for families and carers, including bereavement care
- workforce development.

The NHS Cancer Plan (2000)

This plan heralded a comprehensive approach to the management of cancer encompassing all aspects of the patient pathway including palliative and terminal care. It saw the establishment of cancer networks and, within these, of palliative care networks with dedicated staff to modernise patient pathways and implement new models of care. Palliative care networks were required to engage relevant stakeholders, assess needs, appraise the range of services available and tackle inequity in service provision across geographical areas and across client groups, including those from ethnic minorities.

The NHS Cancer Plan (2000) makes it clear that service care providers are expected to act on and implement formal guidance issued by NICE. Furthermore, all cancer networks were charged with implementing NICE guidance on supportive and palliative care. A formal implementation plan was required by the Department of Health (DoH) from each network in September 2004.

The implications of NICE guidance for patients from South-Asian communities

Guidance on palliative care services has particular implications and importance for patients from ethnic minorities and their families. For example, although there are few reliable sources of data for the prevalence of heart failure amongst different ethnic-minority groups, it is known that people of South-Asian origin have a greater risk of developing coronary artery disease, resulting in part from their high prevalence of obesity and diabetes (NICE Chronic Heart Failure October, 2003).

Since general practitioners are now reimbursed for carrying out regular health assessments of their patients, there are greater incentives to identify life-limited patients, some of whom may be entering their last months. Establishing registers that include patients from South-Asian communities should provide opportunities for clinicians to review individual patients' prognoses and ensure that the care services available to them are matched to their needs instead of assuming that South Asians are a homogenous group who would prefer to 'look after their own'.

This recent NICE guidance applies to all patients with cancer, regardless of ethnic origin. Recommendations are also based on the principle that a patient's identified needs are addressed, irrespective of gender or age. The guidance also makes a number of specific references to the importance of providing patients and their families with written information about available services in appropriate languages. The need to coordinate services to provide seamless and accessible care from the time a patient is first referred up to the end-stage of their life is highlighted.

The guidance further specifically identifies the need to recruit representatives from black and ethnic-minority communities on newly established partnership groups to oversee the development and delivery of cancer services. Underpinning this is the philosophy that patients should be able to access support delivered by people from the same cultural or ethnic group as themselves wherever possible (Koffman and Higginson, 2004). The NICE guidance also recommends that all health and social care professionals should 'undergo diversity or cultural awareness training to promote effective communication with people from ethnic-minority communities'.

Finally, the section on spiritual support services identifies the needs of different faith groups. For example, for some Muslims, the need to identify the direction of Mecca and the recognition of a speedy burial in their tradition are highlighted.

End of life care

At the end of 2003, the then Secretary of State for Health, John Reid, announced an allocation of £12 million across England and Wales to support end-of-life care for cancer patients. The Liverpool Care of the Dying Pathway (*Panel 1.3*); the *Preferred Place of Care* documents (*Panel 1.4*); and the Macmillan Gold Standard Framework (*Panel 1.5*), which is a practice-based framework of care intended for use in the last six to twelve months of a patient's life, have emerged as models of care. There is an expectation that the monies released in 2003 on a recurring basis would be mainstreamed from 2006. However, the Secretary of State for Health has also identified the need to extend palliative care for cancer patients to all other patients suffering from life-limiting illnesses (Finlay *et al*, 2002) and specifically patients dying from chronic obstructive pulmonary disease (COPD), renal disease and heart failure — the last two being of particular relevance to South Asians.

Panel 1.3: The Liverpool Care Pathway (LCP)

The Liverpool Care Pathway (LCP) is a framework of care intended for use in the last forty-eight to seventy-two hours of a patient's life. It can be adapted to any care setting. The tool has been designed as a multi-professional document, which provides an evidence-based framework for end-of-life care. This pathway provides guidance on the different aspects of care required, including comfort measures, anticipatory prescribing of medicines, and discontinuation of inappropriate interventions. In addition, psychological and spiritual care and family support are included.

Panel 1.4: Preferred Place of Care (PPC)

The *Preferred Place of Care* (PPC) document has been designed to facilitate patient choice in end-of-life care. It provides a mechanism for identifying patients' preferences about where they receive care and any specific issues that arise about the care they are receiving. In many cases, patients' initial choices change. The documentation is a method of mapping and analysing these changes so that future care-planning can be informed and targeted to meet individual patients' needs.

Panel 1.5: Gold Standards Framework (GSF)

The Gold Standards Framework is a practice-based framework of care intended for use in the last six to twelve months of a patient's life. It includes the following elements:

- **Communication** — Practices are asked to keep a supportive care register, highlighting details of patients requiring palliative care; carer details; current treatment regimes, etc. They hold monthly palliative-healthcare team meetings to disseminate information within the wider team and ensure a cohesive approach to care. These meetings encourage discussion around psychosocial and physical issues, with the use of forward planning for significant changes in a patient's condition, thus reducing the likelihood of 'panic' admissions to acute settings at the end of life (Costantini and Higginson et *al*, 2003).
- **Coordination** — A person within the palliative-healthcare team acts as coordinator for the supportive care register etc, and is the 'key worker' within the practice for both the patient/carer and other team members to liaise, if any circumstances change. The coordinator should be able to identify if relevant documentation, for example social services referral, has been generated.
- **Control of symptoms** — Regular assessments are undertaken throughout the patient journey, including pain and symptom assessment. The results are documented in the supportive care register and are discussed within the palliative-healthcare team meetings, so that all relevant personnel are up to date with the situation. There are clear guidelines within the assessment tool for when a referral to specialist palliative care might be indicated, eg. if symptoms are unresolved. A quality-of-life assessment tool is also included within the documentation to assess improvements/deterioration in a patient's condition.
- **Continuity out of hours** — Details about a patient's medical status is sent to 'out of hours' providers, so that in the event of being called out to a patient, there is some baseline information on which to make an assessment. If forward planning has taken place, any drugs or equipment required should already be in place within the patient's home.
- **Carer support** — The tool includes a carer's needs assessment, which takes into account the emotional and physical impact of being a carer, and the measures taken to address and support carers. The use of the Marie-Curie nursing service is one method of providing respite, and the tool actively encourages this as part of planned care. Contained within the home care pack is a series of information and contact numbers for various organisations that can provide information and support to people caring for someone at home. Practices are encouraged to devise a bereavement protocol, to include a practice bereavement letter, which contains information about benefits, support services and local contact numbers for families after a patient's death.

Conclusions

In spite of all the legislation cited above, a recent document, *Dying in Older Age* (2005), commissioned by Help the Aged, paints a bleak picture of a future faced by thousands of elderly British as they approach the end of their lives. It reports that although more and more young people with terminal illness are allowed to die at home or in the comfort of a hospice (20%), only 8% of the elderly do so. A further 100,000 pensioners — of whom Asians make up a growing percentage — die in care homes each year, many surrounded by untrained care assistants who lack the skills to communicate with residents or properly assess their needs. Although most patients admit that they would prefer to die at home or in a hospice, a continuing lack of community nurses and resources means their final wish is denied (Edmonds and Rogers, 2003). The report further states that this is a sad reflection of our society, where 'social death' occurs well before physical death.

The success of any legislation will depend on factors such as the individual practitioner's experience and commitment to care; this factor probably accounts for the variable success of care services for all patients, including those from South-Asian communities. The provision of an out-of-hours palliative care service is not adequately addressed by any of the legislation. Continuity of care for all patients is paramount at each stage of their illness. Services should be tailor-made to meet the needs of individual patients including those from minority ethnic communities. This entails dialogue between primary, secondary and tertiary care professionals, including those in hospices, underpinned by a commitment from care providers in partnership with stakeholders.

Key points of *Chapter I*

■ Britain's elderly South-Asian population is growing. There will be a need for greater palliative-care provision.

■ South Asians are not a homogenous group — one should therefore not assume that they will 'look after their own'.

■ At present, diabetes, cardiovascular and renal disease are the main reasons for South Asians requiring palliative care.

■ There is legislation underpinning the following in palliative care:
  ❖ patients should be able to maintain acceptable lifestyles
  ❖ partnerships with community groups should be formed to oversee development and delivery of service
  ❖ there should be diversity and cultural awareness training for healthcare professionals
  ❖ written information should be available on services in appropriate languages.

References

Costantini M, Higginson IJ, Boni L, Orengo MA, Garrone E, Henriquet F, Bruzzi P (2003) Effect of a palliative home care team on hospital admissions among patients with advanced cancer. *Palliat Med* **17**: 315–21

Dobson R (2005) Age discrimination denies elderly people a 'dignified death'. *BMJ* **330**: 1288

Edmonds P (2004) Organisation of palliative care service. *Medicine* **32**: 2–3

Edmonds P, Rogers A (2003) 'If only someone had told me...': a review of the care of patients dying in hospital. *Clin Med* **3**: 149–52

Finlay IG, Higginson IJ, Goodwin DM, Cook AM, Edwards AGK, Hood K, Douglas H-R, Normand C (2002) Palliative care in hospital, hospice, at home: results from a systematic review. *Ann Oncol* **13**: 257–64

Gomes B, Higginson IJ (2004) Home or hospital? Choices at the end of life. *J R Soc Med* **97**: 413–14

Koffman J, Higginson IJ (2004) Dying to be home? Preferred location of death of first-generation black Caribbean and native-born white patients in the United Kingdom. *J Palliat Med* **7**: 628–36

NICE Guideline No. 5 (2003) *Chronic Heart Failure — National Clinical Guideline for Diagnosis and Management in Primary and Secondary Care*

NICE Guidance CG12 (2004) *Chronic Obstructive Pulmonary Disease: Full Guideline*. Published as a supplement to *Thorax*, the journal of the British Thoracic Society

NICE Guidance on Cancer Services (2004) *Improving Supportive and Palliative Care for Adults with Cancer* (the manual)

Developing culturally competent services in palliative care: management perspectives

Paula McGee, Mark RD Johnson

Women who teach [nursing] *in India must know the languages, the religions, superstitions and customs of the women to be taught… it ought to be a truism to say the very same for England.*
Florence Nightingale (1894)

The 2001 population census for the UK shows that 7.9% of a total population of about 58 million people are members of black and other minority ethnic groups. Of these, people from the Indian subcontinent and the Caribbean make up the largest proportions (UK National Statistics Online, www.statistics.gov.uk; *Table 2.1*).

Inclusion of all minorities (recorded in the Census 'Ethnicity' question) raises the proportion of the population who identify themselves as a 'minority' to more than one in eight (12.5%) of the UK population. It is also worth noting that while one in five of the population stated that they had 'no religion' or did not answer the question on religion in the census, over 70% stated that they were Christian and a further 3% gave their religion as Muslim. One person in every hundred was Hindu. In cities such as Leicester, as much as 15% of the population was Hindu and 11% Muslim. There are also significant populations who recorded their faith as Jewish, Sikh or Buddhist. Surveys show that members of minority ethnic groups frequently identify with a religion as well as an ethnic group, and are less likely to say that religious identity is not important (Modood *et al*, 1997).

The 2001 UK census shows the increasing diversity of the UK population, a factor that creates particular challenges for managers in all healthcare services, especially those that are concerned with meeting the needs of people with life-

Table 2.1: Black and ethnic-minority groups in the UK (2001)	
Ethnic-minority group	**Percentage of minority population**
Mixed background	15
Asian/British — Indian	23
Asian/British — Pakistani	16
Asian/British — Bangladeshi	6
Asian/British — Other	5
Black/British — Caribbean	12
Black/British — African	11
Black/British — Other	2
Chinese	5
Other ethnic group(s)	5

Figures rounded to nearest whole number. Total based on 4.6 million, making up 7.9% of UK population. Source: 2001 Census (Crown copyright acknowledged).

limiting illnesses. Easing suffering to enable individuals to live their remaining lives to the full requires a particular skill and commitment, a full understanding of the meaning of care as a concept that ascribes value to others and an approach based on engagement with them in every aspect of life — physical, psychological, social and spiritual. Such engagement includes activities based on 'doing with' or 'doing for' the individual, such as maintaining safety and dignity or providing physical assistance that focuses on being with that person, for example, through emotional support and the complex art of 'presencing' (Benner *et al*, 1996; Benner and Wrubel, 1989). Inherent in all these activities is the need for highly developed clinical and interpersonal skills that can be used to inform empathic, therapeutic relationships between patients and professionals within an environment in which patients, their families and the staff feel that their dignity, rights and well-being are respected and valued.

The increasing diversity of the UK population means that patients and

---

Panel 2.1: Definitions of 'culture' and 'ethnicity' in this chapter

- **Culture** is a learned way of thinking and feeling that is shared with others and which provides a particular way of being in and experiencing the world. It is a type of 'mental software' (Hofstede, 1994).
- **Ethnicity** refers to membership of a socially defined group of people who may be characterised by culture, language, etc. Ethnicity is the ever-changing product of traditions and cultural practices. It is situational and contextual (Culley, 2000).

professionals frequently do not share the same culture, values, beliefs or ethnicity (*Panel 2.1*).

Diversity raises issues about service provision in any healthcare field. But, in palliative care, which is rooted in Western, white, Christian culture, there has until recently been little attempt to create an environment for care that is truly socially inclusive. The creation of this environment is primarily dependent on leaders and managers. Our aim in this chapter is to explore how diversity management and the understanding of the concept of cultural competence by policy-makers can improve heath care, such as palliative care, for South Asians and other minority ethnic groups.

We will begin with an overview of current health policy and legislation that places requirements on healthcare organisations not only to recognise diversity, but also to show how such recognition is enacted. The concept of cultural competence is then outlined in relation to management in palliative care. This is followed by consideration of the key questions to be addressed in the design and delivery of palliative-care services for members of diverse communities.

Policy and legislation

Current health policy aims to improve the health of the population in general, including members of black and other minority ethnic groups who experience inequalities, at least in part, because services do not adequately meet their health needs (Department of Health [DoH], 1997, 2000). There is ample evidence that members of black and minority ethnic groups experience discrimination in health care, both as employees (Beishon *et al*, 1995; Darr, 1998; Klem and Notter, 2001; Notter and Hepburn, 2004) and as patients (DoH, 2003a; Sainsbury Centre for Mental Health, 2002; McGee, 2000). The inquiry into the death of David Bennett, a young black man detained in a mental-health clinic, stated that:

> *at present people from the black and minority ethnic communities... are not getting the service they are entitled to. Putting it bluntly, this is a disgrace. The NHS is national.*
>
> Norfolk, Suffolk and Cambridgeshire
> Strategic Health Authority (NSCSHA, 2003)

These inquiries unequivocally report that institutional racism is as prevalent in the NHS as in other public services. The term 'institutional racism' was coined in the inquiry into the notorious death of another young black man, Stephen Lawrence, and defined as 'the collective failure of an organisation to provide an appropriate and professional service to people because of their colour, culture or ethnic origin' (Home Office, 1999: para 6.4). Institutional racism is thus a result of organisational processes, procedures and structures that have the effect of discriminating against members of black and minority ethnic groups even though individual members of staff may not do so. Ignorance of cultural or religious beliefs and ethnic differences, intolerance, stereotypical ideas and prejudices can all contribute to the development and maintenance of institutional racism that is enacted through, for example, the inappropriate timing of services, lack of physical access and negative staff attitudes that serve to exclude members of black and other minority ethnic groups.

Current health policy and recent changes in UK legislation can be seen as strategies that aim to bring about cultural change in all aspects of the health service. One example is the Protection from Harassment Act (1997) which provides for the introduction of an action plan, by the DoH, to adopt a zero-tolerance approach in protecting employees from violence and aggression in the workplace and, in particular, to make clear to patients, relatives, staff and the public in general that racial harassment is now considered unacceptable (DoH, 1998). Prior to this, numerous research reports had shown the extent of the problem (Beishon *et al*, 1995; NAHA, 1988; Darr, 1998; Gerrish *et al*, 1996) and, disappointingly, have continued to do so (Notter and Hepburn, 2004; NSCSHA, 2003; McGee, 2000). Nevertheless, this action plan represents an organisational commitment to change, led by those in the most senior positions in the service through the explicit statement of values and the ways in which these are to be enacted.

A second example of an attempt at cultural change is evident in the Race Relations (Amendment) Act (2000). This renders institutional racism illegal and provides for the mandatory development of race-equality schemes in all parts of the public sector, including health. The aim of these schemes is to:

- Propel diversity into the main management arena through the requirements placed on managers in each organisation.
- Critically appraise policies and procedures for evidence of discriminatory practices.
- Consult with members of the minority ethnic groups in the locality regarding the need for change and the specific changes required.
- Implement and publicise the outcomes.
- Provide staff development to facilitate change.

Added impetus was given to this move, in the health service, by the announcement of a 'ten point plan' for race equality by the Chief Executive of the NHS in February 2004 (Crisp, 2004). This laid out five targets in service delivery and five in human resource management, making it clear that both were intimately linked (*Table 2.2*).

Such requirements move well beyond previous policies such as equal opportunities towards diversity management. Equal-opportunities policy focuses mainly on non-discrimination and the differential distribution of opportunity. The concept of equal opportunities dictates that everyone should receive the same services, at the same standard, irrespective of the ethnic group to which they belong. But notions of rights and legal compliance tend to cast equal opportunities outside the mainstream of management concerns (Cornelius, 2002). By contrast, diversity management focuses on differences, promoting equality through understanding and respecting these differences.

Table 2.2: Targets in service delivery and human resources management

Health services and outcomes
■ Strategic direction
■ Align incentives
■ Development
■ Communication
■ Partnership
Developing people
■ Mentoring
■ Leadership action
■ Expand training, development/career opportunities
■ Systematic tracking
■ Celebrate Achievements

Source: Race Equality Action Plan (DoH, 2004).

The application of diversity management principles in health care has touched management priorities in a more strategic way than equal opportunities. For example, diversity management has enabled services to respond to demographic shifts through strategies aimed at recruiting and retaining members of minority groups into the workforce (Cornelius, 2002).

This change in emphasis has several implications for managers of palliative-care services. First, palliative care has developed in association with Western Christian cultural and religious values (Gaffin *et al*, 1996) and was initially a service in which care was provided by and for a predominantly white population (in common, it must be said, with much of the NHS). Therefore, the whole terminology and ethos of hospital care has strong links to Christian religious institutions. Diversity management requires:

■ Expansion of values and beliefs that underpin modern palliative care to include those of other traditions.
■ An understanding of the fact that, although care is a universal phenomenon, members of each culture have particular ideas about what constitutes appropriate care and what does not (Leininger and McFarland, 2002). For example, in Western cultures, if a family member other than one's immediate relative, is unwell, it may be sufficient to send a 'Get Well Soon' card and some flowers. People tend to stay away to allow the individual time to recover. In cultures that originate in countries without

a welfare state, this would typically be considered very uncaring because it is the (extended) family's responsibility to help members who are ill. In other words, people demonstrate care by visiting rather than staying away. However, this may cause problems for the managers of hospices and hospitals, where large numbers of visitors are seen as a 'problem' (Firth, 2001; Faull *et al*, 1998).

- Diversity management in this context requires a cultural shift towards a more inclusive approach that challenges stereotypical thinking, such as the belief that members of black and other minority ethnic groups will always be cared for at home and by family members. This has often led to a failure to offer care service support to minority families (Murray and Brown, 1998). Even where such care is truly preferred, carers will need respite and support from services that they can trust to look after the patient in an appropriate way.

- A patient-focused approach is to be retained but expanded to take account of diverse cultural values about decision-making and responsibility. Service providers need to understand that clinical and technical competence is not enough, as palliative care has always placed the patient at the centre of activity. Furthermore, professionals in that field should seek to work in partnership with individuals, recognising that the true nature of care lies not in technical or clinical competence, but the way in which these are delivered. In adopting this patient-focused approach, palliative care should promote the idea of concordance — ie. negotiating to provide care that the patient both needs and wants (DoH, 2003b).

- The development of a workforce that reflects the diversity within the population served and a working environment in which members of black and other minority ethnic groups can feel valued.

All of these notions may be summarised as requiring an organisation to move beyond a narrow technical, specialist ability to perform its basic functions to a broader and more inclusive understanding of cultural competence.

Cultural competence

Cultural competence is an evolving process that depends on self-awareness, knowledge and skills. It begins with an acceptance of differences, each of which is applicable to the organisation as a whole and to the individuals who work within it. It may also be seen as operating at three levels:

- developing self-awareness
- knowledge
- development and application of skills.

Developing self-awareness

Developing self-awareness is the first level of cultural competence. It requires all those working in palliative care to examine the ways in which their own behaviour, attitudes and beliefs may help or hinder their dealings with patients and their families. From a management perspective, this involves reviewing the organisational culture and re-conceptualising its values, beliefs, policies and procedures in terms of commitment to diversity management. Embedding the race-equality strategy into the formal organisational culture is an important step but, if it is to be more than just a paper exercise, managers must also examine ways in which they can bring about change in organisational culture and enable staff to develop their own individual self-awareness. This requires managers to consider the existing organisational style in communicating with staff and users, and the subtle ways in which current systems may perpetuate institutional racism.

For staff, self-awareness also leads to an appraisal of different styles of communication that may be culturally or linguistically determined (Campinha Bacote, 2003). For example, in Hindi, the most commonly spoken South-Asian language, a patient may say 'mera dil me dard hai'. Now, in strictly literal terms, this means 'my heart is hurting', but its more common meaning is simply 'I am upset'. An understanding of the patient's usual or preferred communication style, coupled with an awareness of one's own, is an essential part of establishing effective communication and the basis for therapeutic relationships.

Far more difficult, in relation to self-awareness, is the issue of attitudes, beliefs and prejudices. No one is immune to having prejudices, but what matters in this context is an awareness of them and the ways in which they may interfere with the care of patients. Acknowledging one's prejudices can be a difficult task, both for an organisation and for individuals, but there are good examples in the literature that can act as guides. One example is the work of Sands and Hale (1988) who argued that there is a culture of poverty that includes not only members of black and other minority ethnic groups, but also elderly people, alcoholics, substance-abusers, the poor and many others who, for one reason or another, have limited means to maintain themselves, cope with people whom they perceive as being in authority, or have little power to exercise their own rights. Such individuals are frequently dehumanised and regarded as inferior by professionals. In this, we can see echoes of the old division between the 'deserving' and 'undeserving' poor — originally codified in the English 'Poor

Law' of 1601 — a concept still evident in the early versions of the welfare state (Callinicos and Jenkins, 1995).

It is through this process of dehumanisation that stereotypes, prejudices and racism develop. However, the use of guided personal contact between individual students and those living in the culture of poverty can do much to offset and challenge such negativity (McGee, 1992). The skills of reflection are crucial to the success of such contact and require the 'investment of time and commitment to establishing and pursuing meaningful dialogue' (Kavanagh *et al*, 1999) to facilitate an attitudinal shift in which both parties move from characterising each other as 'them' (the Other) towards 'X, whom we know' (Us). Part of achieving this shift involves a recognition of the ways in which providers of palliative care represent to patients the culture and the power of the health service in which they are employed, and the ways in which that power and culture can create and sustain inequalities (Papps and Ramsden, 1996).

Knowledge

Knowledge is the second level in developing cultural competence (Campinha Bacote, 2003). In itself, knowledge will not facilitate culturally competent palliative-care provision, but it is needed to inform both managers and practitioners about appropriate codes of behaviour. From a management perspective, developing an appropriate knowledge-base begins with application of ethnic monitoring that is geared to identifying the diverse elements in the population to be served. In palliative care, these data should include information about such factors as the culture, ethnicity, religion and also preferred language of those who use current services and epidemiological data about the types of problems for which they require care (Johnson, 2001). Such a database should also include information about black and minority ethnic groups in the locality whose members do not appear to use palliative care services as a prelude to establishing why this may be so.

Absence of data by ethnic group is itself a barrier to improving access to palliative care — but absence of evidence of use is not absence of need. Reducing inequalities is dependent on information that allows measurement of the severity of health problems, the need for and appropriateness of treatments and the outcomes obtained. This has been made more difficult by a dearth of good-quality ethnic data in relation to many issues, including incidence of cancer in older members of black and other minority ethnic groups (Johnson *et al*, 2001; Aspinall and Jacobson, 2004).

For staff, developing knowledge should, initially at least, focus on the particular black and minority ethnic groups represented in the locality in relation to their ideas about the body, health, illness, treatment and care.

Beliefs about these factors are culturally determined. For example, the causes of illness and disease are frequently conceptualised in terms of relationships, either between the individual and other people, or between that person and God. Thus, practitioners need to understand a patient's frame of reference in answering questions such as 'why me?' (Helman, 2000). Similarly, ideas about the body may differ. For instance, some South-Asian people have no concept of the circulation of the blood (personal communication: Gatrad, 2005) and, therefore, no words to describe it. In such circumstances, explaining conditions such as diabetes or peripheral vascular disease, as shown in an Australian study (Trudgen, 2000), presents the practitioner with a number of challenges.

Notions of the ways in which illness should be treated, the type of treatment and the way in which the professionals should behave are all part of the knowledge-base of the culturally competent practitioner. However, practitioners — be they doctors, nurses or allied health professionals — must also acknowledge that this knowledge-base can only ever be partial. It is through encounters with patients that knowledge will be extended, provided of course that the practitioner keeps an open mind and recognises that individual preferences and differences matter more than generalisations (Kai, 2003).

Development and application of skills

Development and application of skills, underpinned by knowledge and self-awareness, is the third level of cultural competence (Campinha Bacote, 2003). From a management perspective, these skills are concerned with tackling institutional racism and ensuring that the criteria for organisational procedures and decisions are clear and equitably applied within the context of a diverse workforce and patient population (Cornelius, 2002). For staff, the development and application of skills is focused on the adaptation of practice in ways that take account of cultural and religious values. For example, some may wish to avoid medication derived from animals because of cultural, religious or secular beliefs. There is little research on this subject, but one small study of Muslim patients found that over half would stop taking prescribed medication if they thought it was of porcine (pig) origin and thus, in their view, haraam — forbidden (Bashir *et al*, 2001). Therefore, exploring patients' beliefs in accordance with the 'patient choice' agenda (DoH, 2003) is important as a basis for achieving concordance.

Paula McGee, Mark RD Johnson

Organisational approaches

It is clearly not enough to examine only the attitudes, knowledge and behaviour of individuals. Managers need to examine the degree to which their services have the commitment, structures and information available to support change. Increasingly, in order to generate the Race Equality Action Plans required under the Race Relations Amendment Act (2001), organisations are turning to the use of toolkits and checklists to examine their whole practice (Chirico *et al*. 2000). Key questions that they need to ask include reviewing the language and 'feel' of the organisation, the data on potential and actual users (monitoring), the mission and management agenda (ensuring that these are designed to be inclusive), staffing, and the overall processes at work, to ensure that these are not unintentionally discriminatory simply because no-one has thought about the degree to which they may be culturally sensitive (or insensitive). In short, managers and board members need to ask themselves and their organisations seven key questions (*Panel 2.2*).

Panel 2.2: Key questions for developing culturally competent mangers in palliative care

- Whom are we here to serve?
- Who are our users?
- Who does what?
- How are users involved?
- How do we work with others?
- Do we respect and celebrate diversity?
- Do we respect and value our staff?

The first key question is to examine whether a needs assessment and profile of the potential users has been undertaken; this should clearly include information from census and surveys about the ethnic and cultural make-up of the catchment area. Following on from this is a need to determine who actually uses the services, and how they come to know about, or be referred to, them. Ethnic monitoring is now well established as a technique, but often the data are collected and never analysed or used; this wastes resources and causes frustration (Johnson 2001).

A clear understanding of responsibilities and the importance of having and implementing policies and protocols is essential. It is best if a 'lead' on matters such as equality and sensitivity is shown and owned by senior managers, rather than left to somebody (else). Designated responsibilities need to be embedded in structures and job roles, so that if a member of staff or director leaves, the impetus for change and monitoring is not lost.

User engagement is now regarded as a fundamental element of all health and social care (and business) planning and management; it is important to ensure that this includes minority communities, even if they are not seen to be using the service at present. This may be made easier by seeking collaborative working arrangements and partnerships with community-based organisations such as religious and social groups. In the process, people in the organisation, and the agency itself, may come to appreciate the value and interest of diverse cultures. Last, but not least, is the need to recruit, respect and support staff from minority backgrounds, which increases the pool of people available to work in the organisation and brings in new and useful skills.

Conclusions

In this chapter, we have explored what is meant by 'diversity', and some of the dimensions that make up this concept. There are now a number of factors that drive the need to pay greater attention to diversity management, including not only commercial good sense, which is still necessary in charitable and statutory bodies as well as in businesses that seek to make a profit, but also legal and moral considerations. We have sought to embed a response to all of these needs in a structure of organisational cultural competence, and laid out a possible pattern or template for managers to address in an audit of their policies and practices. This includes a seven step approach to review what is being done, at not only the level of overall structure and policy, but also in terms of everyday activity, service development and staff training. Clearly, all of these steps can be seen to be good in themselves, and not simply beneficial in respect of ethnic, racial, religious or cultural diversity. A point we are seeking to make is that cultural competence is a good professional and organisational practice, which will benefit the whole organisation and all of its users. By paying attention to detail, and examining the degree to which issues of diversity are addressed, a cultural competence audit will uncover many other areas where the organisation may not be functioning optimally.

Key points of *Chapter 2*

- Increasing diversity of the UK population challenges professionals to provide services that are truly socially inclusive.
- Current health policy is intended to reduce health inequalities through the provision of accessible and appropriate services and by tackling racial discrimination through diversity management.
- Diversity management requires an expansion of the values and attitudes that underpin palliative care to ensure that service provision is truly patient-centred.
- Cultural competence is an evolving process that depends on knowledge, self-awareness and the adaptation of skills.
- Cultural competence is an essential part of professional practice in all disciplines involved in palliative care.
- Organisations, such as hospices and NHS trusts, also need to develop cultural competence in:
  - ❖ meeting the healthcare needs of members of diverse communities in their localities
  - ❖ developing and managing a palliative care workforce that reflects the diversity of the local population
  - ❖ creating a care environment in which both patients and staff from diverse backgrounds feel valued and safe.

References

Aspinall PJ, Jacobson B (2004) *Ethnic Disparities in Health and Health Care: a Focused Review of the Evidence and Selected Examples of Good Practice*. London Health Observatory, London

Bashir A, Asif F, Lacey F, Langley C, Marrior J, Wilson K (2001) Concordance in Muslim patients in primary care. *Int J Pharm Practice* **9**(Suppl): R78

Beishon S, Virdee S, Hagell A (1995) *Nursing in a Multi-ethnic NHS*. Policy Studies Institute, London

Benner P, Wrubel J (1989) *The Primacy of Caring: Stress and Coping in Health and Illness*. Addison Wesley Publishing Company, Menlo Park, California

Benner P, Tanner C, Chesla C (1996) *Expertise in Nursing Practice: Caring, Clinical Judgement and Ethics*. Springer Publishing Company, New York

Callinicos A, Jenkins G (1995) Community without Care: Socialist Review 186 (http://pubs.socialistreviewindex.org.uk/sr186/callinicos.htm)

(accessed 5 May 2005)

Campinha-Bacote J (2003) *The Process of Cultural Competence in the Delivery of Healthcare Services: a Culturally Competent Model of Care.* 4th edn. Available from Transcultural Care Associates at http://www.transculturalcare.net (accessed May 2005)

Chirico S, Johnson M, Pawar A, Scott M (2000) *The Toolbox: Culturally Competent Organisations, Services and Care Pathways.* Bedfordshire Health Promotion Agency, Bedford

Cornelius C (ed) (2002) *Building Workplace Equality: Ethics, Diversity and Inclusion.* Thompson, London

Crisp N (2004) Race Equality Action Plan. Available at http://www.dh.gov.uk/PublicationsAndStatistics (accessed May 2005)

Culley L, Dyson S (eds) (2001) *Ethnicity and Nursing Practice.* Palgrave, Basingstoke

Darr A (1998) *Improving the Recruitment and Retention of Asian Students in Nursing: Midwifery, Radiography and Physiotherapy Courses: a Qualitative Research Study.* Report available from the University of Bradford School of Health Studies, Bradford

DoH (1997) *The NHS: Modern and Dependable.* DoH, London

DoH (1998) *Tackling Racial Harassment in the NHS: a Plan for Action.* DoH, Wetherby

DoH (2000) *The NHS Plan: a Plan for Investment, a Plan for Reform.* DoH, London

DoH (2003) *Building on the Best: Choice, Responsiveness and Equity in the NHS.* DoH, London

DoH (2003a) *Delivering Race Equality: a Framework for Action.* Mental Health Services consultation document. DoH, London

DoH (2003b) *Choice, Responsiveness and Equity in the NHS and Social Care.* A national consultation. DoH, London

Faull C, Carter Y, Woof R (eds) (1998) *Handbook of Palliative Care.* Blackwell, Oxford

Firth S (2001) *Wider Horizons: Care of the Dying in a Multicultural Society.* National Council for Hospice and Specialist Palliative Care Services, London

Gaffin J, Hill D, Penso D (1996) Opening doors: improving access to hospice and specialist palliative care services by members of the black and minority ethnic communities. *Br J Cancer* (Suppl)**29**: S51–S53

Gerrish K, Husband C, Mackenzie J (1996) *Nursing for a Multi-ethnic Society.* Open University Press, Buckinghamshire

Helman C (2000) *Culture, Health and Illness*. 4th edn. Heinemann Butterworth, Oxford

Hofstede G (1994) *Culture and Organisations: Software of the Mind: Intercultural Co-operation and its Importance for Survival*. HarperCollins, London

Home Office (1999) *The Stephen Lawrence Inquiry: Report of an Inquiry by Sir William Macpherson of Cluny*. The Stationery Office, London

Johnson MRD (2001) Ethnic monitoring and nursing. In: Culley L, Dyson S (eds) *Ethnicity and Nursing Practice*. Palgrave, Basingstoke

Johnson MRD, Bains J, Chauhan J, Saleem B, Tomlins R (2001) *Improving Palliative Care for Minority Ethnic Communities in Birmingham: a Report for Birmingham Specialist Community Health NHS Trust and Macmillan Cancer Relief*. Mary Seacole Research Centre, Leicester (available as Seacole Working Paper 5: www.dmu.ac.uk/msrc)

Kai J (ed) (2003) *Ethnicity, Health and Primary Care*. Oxford University Press, Oxford

Kavanagh K, Absalom K, Bell W, Schliessman I (1999) Connecting and becoming culturally competent: a Lakota example. *Adv Nurs Sci* **21**(3): 13

Klem R, Notter J (2002) *The Recruitment and Retention in Nursing and Professions Allied to Medicine of Individuals from Black and Minority Ethnic Communities*. Report published by the Faculty of Health and Community Care, University of Central England, Birmingham

Leininger M, McFarland M (2002) *Transcultural Nursing: Concepts, Theories, Research and Practice*. 3rd edn. McGraw-Hill, New York

McGee P (1992) *Teaching Transcultural Care*. Chapman and Hall, London

McGee P (2000) Culturally Sensitive Nursing: a Critique. Unpublished PhD Thesis. University of Central England, Birmingham

Modood T, Berthoud R, Lakey J, Nazroo J, Smith P, Virdee S, Beishon S (1997) *Ethnic Minorities in Britain: Diversity and Disadvantage*. PSI Report 843. Policy Studies Institute, London

Murray U, Brown D (1998) *They Look After Their Own, Don't They? Inspection of Community Care Services for Black and Minority Older People*. DoH Social Care Group and Social Services Inspectorate, London

National Association of Health Authorities (1988) *Action not Words: a Strategy to Improve Health Services for Black and Minority Ethnic Groups*. NAHA, Birmingham

Norfolk, Suffolk and Cambridgeshire Strategic Health Authority (2003) *Independent Inquiry into the Death of David Bennett*. Report of an inquiry set up under HSG (94)27. Chaired by Sir John Blofeld, Cambridge NSCSHA, Cambridge

Notter J, Hepburn B (2004) *Improving the Representation of Black and Minority Ethnic Staff within the Ambulance Services.* Report published by the Faculty of Health and Community Care, University of Central England, Birmingham

Papps E, Ramsden I (1996) Cultural safety in nursing: the New Zealand experience. *Int J Qual Health Care* **8**(5): 491–7

Sainsbury Centre for Mental Health (2002) *Breaking the Circles of Fear: a Review of the Relationship between Mental Health Services and African and Caribbean Communities.* Sainsbury Centre for Mental Health, London

Sands R, Hale S (1988) Enhancing cultural sensitivity in clinical practice. *J Natl Black Nurses Assoc* **2**(1): 54–63

Trudgen R (2000) *Why Warriors Lie Down and Die: Towards an Understanding of Why the People of Arnhem Land Face the Greatest Crisis in Health and Education since European Contact.* Aboriginal Resource and Development Services Inc, Darwin, Australia

UK 2001 Census. Available at http://www.statistics.gov.uk (accessed May 2005)

Section Two:
A Question Of Faith

The language of religious symbolism: rendering visible the invisible

Sabina Gatrad, Rashid Gatrad

The worst moment of an atheist is when he feels grateful but does not know who to thank.
Wendy Ward

Our experiences suggest that whilst many clinicians understand the religious symbols (albeit often unknowingly) of the dominant Judeo-Christian traditions, they are less likely to know the symbols of other religions. It is therefore important briefly to explore the philosophy underpinning religious symbols and rituals that are so often of considerable importance to people from South-Asian backgrounds, particularly towards the end of life. In so doing, it is hoped that caregivers will develop their own professional understanding of these issues and accordingly support their patients with life-limiting illnesses.

Most Muslims, Hindus and Sikhs will remain secure in their faith in the face of adversity, but this does not mean that they will not ask existential questions. Understandably, patients and their families may examine their beliefs even more deeply in times of crisis, searching for a reason for what is happening to them. But this need not distract them from the unshakeable beliefs they hold, central to which is a belief in God, and which is often manifested through the use of religious symbols.

Such symbols for millions of South Asians around the world are not an aside or a theory — they are fundamental to who they are and their whole way of life. All major religions teach that physical death is not the end; in this regard, symbols help alleviate spiritual pain and find hope that extends beyond physical life. Therefore, engaging through symbols on a spiritual quest and examining personal beliefs and doubts does not distract the religious pilgrim from the core tenet of his or her faith, but helps cement it.

It is in times of celebration and tragedy that symbols give meaning to moments of intense experience. They are thought to provide a calming effect in difficult situations, ranging from the care of a very sick newborn baby to palliative care of the elderly. Through the use of symbols and artefacts, such as statues amongst Hindus, concepts are represented in graphical compositions. Images range between those that are like pictures through to abstract images that can be combined to form syntax — for example, a holy picture, scarred by years of being folded in a pocket, or prayer beads that have been handed down for generations within a family. Whatever the visual or tactile qualities of the symbol, the value is in the meaning it has for the person to whom it belongs.

Panel A: Two examples of the importance of religious symbols

A terminal elderly Hindu patient was delighted when the statue of Vishnu (one of the Hindu gods) was brought into his room. 'Now I am at peace with myself — I know that I am at one with my God — and am ready for what my new world will offer me,' he was heard saying.

Similarly, a young Muslim mother who had lost two premature babies was very grateful that the Tawiz (black string) attached to her new baby son's wrist was not disturbed or removed during the insertion of an intravenous line, for it contained holy scriptures and was worn to ward off evil.

Panel B: Some examples of religious symbols

- *Muslims* — prayer beads; Tawiz (a black string with religious scriptures attached to it); burning of joss sticks.
- *Hindus* — statues of gods and the burning of a lit lamp called Diva.
- *Sikhs* — five Ks (see *Chapter 8*) on or around them; pictures of Gurus (religious figures).

Symbols can give a sense of purpose and make a big difference to whether a person feels in control. Ill people will find strength in feeling comfortable in their surroundings and to be confident that those who care for them understand something about their faith and its symbolic nature (*Panel A*).

Symbols come in different forms. A Hindu lady may have a Bindi (red dot) on her forehead; a Muslim may have a beard and a Topi (skull cap); and, among other symbols, a Sikh may wear a turban and a Kara (steel bangle) (*Panel B*).

The ways in which prayers are conducted by some adherents of South-Asian religious traditions in the form of recitation and rhythm during worship are also of course deeply symbolic.

It is very easy to provide religious symbols to patients and pay lip-service to the idea of improving the quality of experiences, particularly of the dying. Encouraging families to bring religious symbols and artefacts into hospital means that carers must undertake training on faith and cultural aspects of care. We believe that training is much more likely to be effective if a 'whole staff' approach is taken. This does not imply that all staff need to be trained in the same way, but that everybody should share a common understanding of the purpose so that implementation extends beyond tokenism.

Where palliative-care services include teams led by bilingual health workers, this can provide greater insight into the needs of South-Asian service users. Furthermore, where patients and their families contribute to discussions about their needs, it is far more likely that care will be matched to individual needs. Considerable trust and support is required if this kind of approach is to be successful. Only then can it truly be said that care is a collaborative partnership in practice.

Conclusions

To healthcare professionals in Europe and the West, some South-Asian beliefs may seem alien or, at best, quaint. Being familiar with South-Asian religious symbols, however, is likely to breed understanding and nurture respect. In contrast, ignorance can create assumptions that may be wildly at variance with the truth. It is important for carers, therefore, to take time to learn about and understand not just practices, but why they are carried out.

It does not always follow that because patients come from a certain ethnic origin, they practise a faith. Some people may wish to maintain practices that are important to them, whilst others express only a nominal allegiance to their faith and are not concerned with orthodox practice. We believe that this tendency will increase with the slow process of acculturation as a result of Western models of schooling and the influences of the media and workplace. Through entering into a dialogue with those who live and breathe different traditions, we hope carers and clinicians will reach a deeper understanding of the needs of those approaching the end of their lives. Living life in the shadow of death is fraught with uncertainties, but when people are able to reflect on important dimensions of the life they have lived — for example, through the use of symbols — they are helped to find meaning that is consistent with their identity.

Sabina Gatrad, Rashid Gatrad

Key points of *Introductory comment*

- Religious symbols are important to Muslims, Hindus and Sikhs.
- Religious symbols may help in calming a patient and alleviating spiritual pain.
- Healthcare professionals should be proactive with the family in the provision of religious symbols.
- There should be a designated space for holy water.

CHAPTER 3

The Muslim grand narrative

Sabina Gatrad, Rashid Gatrad, Aziz Sheikh

To each is a goal to which God turns him; then strive together (as in a race) towards all that is good. Wheresoever ye are, God will bring you together. For God Hath power over all things.
Qur'an 2: 148

Although religions are diverse, they share a claim to divine inspiration and the imparting of moral truths and guidance passed down through generations. Such beliefs, prayers, symbols and ceremony can help religious communities and the individuals within them in times of celebration and tragedy. To the uninitiated, these practices may seem rigid, but for those within the tradition they are symbolic and hold deep meaning. In this and the following chapter, we will explore what gives meaning to such moments of intense human experience for Muslims. In the first of three narratives of South-Asian religions, we seek to share an 'insider's view' of Islam in the context of palliative care. We believe that, for the reasons shown in *Panel 3.1*, narratives are an excellent way of engaging, exploring and sharing experience with healthcare professionals.

Panel 3.1: Attributes of narratives (adapted from Greenhalgh et al, 2005)

- Stories are a natural and universal form of communication.
- Stories are sense-making devices — they allow people to make sense of events and actions and link them to past experience.
- Stories embrace complexity — they can capture all the elements of a problem.
- Stories offer insight into what might (or could or should) have been, and hence consider different options and their likely endings.
- Stories have an ethical dimension, and hence motivate learning.
- Stories occur in both formal and informal space. Hence, story-based learning can occur from a very wide range of sources.
- Stories are performative. They focus attention on actions (and inactions) and provide lessons on how action could change in future situations.

Table 3.1: Muslims in the UK by country of birth (Maria O'Beirne, 2004)

Country	Percentage %
UK and Ireland	31
Europe	3
Middle East	6
Africa	8
Indian Subcontinent	43
Asia	1
Other	8

Globally, there are an estimated one billion Muslims (Gatrad and Sheikh, 2005), forming one fifth of the world's population. There are 1.6 million Muslims in the UK (Census, 2001), of which over 40% are from India, Pakistan and Bangladesh; most of the rest come from the Middle East, North Africa and eastern Europe (*Table 3.1*).

Though ethnically heterogeneous, all these diverse communities are tied up by a religious narrative that has permeated almost all aspect of Muslim culture (Winter, 2000). The term Muslim defines one who has freely submitted him or herself to the will of Allah (God). Muslims follow the religion of Islam which is, in its current manifestation, over 1400 years old. The word Islam means 'peace', which is acquired through submission to the will of God. The Islamic holy book, the Qur'an, was revealed to Prophet Muhammad (may God's peace and blessings be on him), the last of the messengers of God and the pinnacle of creation. The guides sent previously included those from the Judeo-Christian traditions such as Abraham, David, Solomon Moses and Jesus (may God's peace and blessings be on them). Muslims hold these prophets, and many more besides, in the highest possible esteem. An appreciation of this may allow Christian chaplains to focus on commonality of beliefs when delivering spiritual care to their Muslim patients.

The five pillars of Islam

The Shahadah or testimony of faith is the declaration that states that, 'There is no deity, but God and that Muhammad is His messenger'. The recitation and therefore reaffirmation of this credal statement is important for Muslims at all times, particularly when in the throes of death.

The term Salah, denoting the five daily prayers, is derived from an Arabic verb which means 'to connect'. This is therefore the very act of communing directly with God. The timings of these prayers vary with the natural cycle of day and night:

- Fajr — before sunrise
- Zuhr — after noon
- Asr — late afternoon
- Maghrib — after sunset
- Isha — late at night.

The prerequisites for Salah are a purity of intention, cleanliness of the body, clothes and environment. A ritual washing in running water, called Wudu, is a prerequisite to any prayer but can be substituted with a dry ablution using dust, if circumstances demand. Although there is a physical element of standing, bending and sitting, these prayers can be performed on the bed whilst sitting or, in the case of the very ill or infirm, with symbolic movements of the eyes.

Zakah, a tax of 2.5% of one's profit, is due to the poor. This helps ensure that all members of society are able to realise their basic needs. A man or woman is a trustee to all that is God's wealth and is therefore accountable to Him. A patient may be anxious about not having fulfilled this duty prior to death.

Sawm or fasting involves abstinence from food, drink and sex from dawn to dusk for a period of a month. The ill and the infirm are excused from this obligation although in reality some patients receiving palliative care may still persist in trying to fulfil this rite. The fasting period ends with a festival called Eid-ul-fitr.

Hajj, the annual pilgrimage to Mecca in Saudi Arabia, should be performed once in a lifetime by those in good health and who can afford it. It represents a celebration of the Patriarch Abraham's readiness to sacrifice his son Ishmael. Some terminally ill Muslims may wish to visit Mecca in the hope of dying there. The end of the pilgrimage, which is a ceremony lasting five days, is marked by another celebration called Eid-ul-adha.

As the Islamic calendar is lunar (355 days), the precise Gregorian calendar dates of Ramadan and the Hajj seasons, and consequently the timing of the two Eids, alters every year by about ten days. Healthcare professionals need to appreciate that a particular Eid may be the last for a terminal patient and many will thus wish to spend this occasion in the company of friends and family.

The sacred law of Islam (Shariah)

Shariah has three main sources:

- The Qur'an. The direct word of God.
- The Hadith (plural Ahadith). The way Prophet Muhammad conducted his life is represented in the form of scriptures called Ahadith. To follow a prophetic tradition is called a Sunnah, examples of which include being circumcised, the sporting of a beard for males and using wood from the Salvadora Persica tree for cleaning teeth (Johnstone, 1998).
- Ijtihad, or the law of deductive logic, underpins the two sources described above and is crucial to the contemporary interpretation and application of sacred law. It is this process of Ijtihad that allows the framing of responses to issues not directly covered in the Qur'an and Sunnah — issues such as whether or not to withhold treatment in a terminally ill patient, for example.

It needs to be noted that since Islam has at least five widely recognised schools of jurisprudence — four within the dominant Sunni tradition (Hanafi, Hanbali, Maliki and Shafi) and one (Jafiri) in the Shi'a tradition — differences in opinions on any given matter are not uncommon. This heterogeneity of views, described by Prophet Muhammad himself as 'a mercy from God', can, if not appreciated, lead to confusion on the part of those trying to understand the range of Islamic rulings on an issue such as cleanliness, for example.

There is no clergy or sacraments in Islam, the only religious authority being the Ulemas (learned men and women trained in highly respected Islamic institutions such as the Al-Azhar University in Cairo). Ethical dilemma are often debated by these scholars and they, by increasingly working in conjunction with specialists from relevant disciplines, reach a consensus edict or Fatwa. Depending on the problem and its interpretation, there may, as alluded to above, be a difference of opinion between different schools of jurisprudence. For example, there is a recognised difference of opinion between the Hanafi school of thinking, which is predominant in South Asia, and others such as the Hanbali school of thinking, more common in Arabia, on the legitimacy of donating and receiving organs for transplantation; the latter are generally in favour, whereas the former object (Gatrad, 1994). It is therefore not unusual for sharply contrasting rulings to coexist. In such circumstances, individuals are generally free to choose whichever ruling they perceive to be closest to the 'truth'.

Halal and Haram

Halal is that which is permitted ie. matters with respect to which no restriction exists. These lawful actions are those that are almost universally acknowledged to be healthy or wholesome — for example, the giving of charity or the institution of marriage. Conversely, Haram refers to matters that God deems to be unhealthy either to individuals or society or both, and has thus forbidden. Examples of Haram acts or states of being include envy, avarice and dishonesty. The general ruling in sacred law is that 'all is allowed except that which is prohibited': law is thus meant, if correctly understood, to be liberating and not restrictive. Therefore, there can be a concession if exceptional circumstances prevail.

The concept of Halal and Haram is part of the total legal system of Islam, the Shariah, and applies to all aspects of life, including marriage, dealings in business, and eating and drinking, to take but a few common examples. The eating of pork is well known to be prohibited or Haram, but less widely appreciated is that adultery, transactions involving the paying or receiving of interest (which is considered exploitative) and suicide are also classed as Haram. For the ill, the consumption of Haram substances may, however, become lawful if circumstances change — for example, if someone's life depended on a certain porcine-derived medication. In the case of no suitable alternative being available, most jurists would rule that the taking of the medication was lawful, if not mandatory (Al-Qaradawi, 1985: 51):

> *But if one is compelled by necessity, neither craving nor transgression — there is on him no sin, for God is Clement, Merciful.*
>
> Qur'an 16: 117

Analgesia and euthanasia

Islam has made human life sacred and has safeguarded its preservation. Because the human race constitutes a single family, an offence against any of its members is an offence against humanity (Al-Qaradawi, 1985: 323). Euthanasia will therefore be regarded as an affront against both the inviolability of human life and society as a whole. For alleviation of pain, Muslim jurists recognise the 'doctrine of double effect', whereby, in the process of analgesia, death may be hastened. This is based on the central teaching that 'actions are to be judged by their intentions'. Therefore, nobody is authorised to end life deliberately, whether one's own or that of another. Withdrawal of food and drink to hasten death is similarly therefore not allowed. Islamic belief is that the time of death is a matter of divine decree and that humans should not be allowed to tamper with this.

Muslims categorically reject Grayling's view (2005) that argues, 'not only does the right to die have a moral basis in the right to a good life but also that choosing when and how to die, should be left to individual choice' through, for example, a living will. For Muslims, such thinking in relation to euthanasia is anathema. The future possibility of doctors being empowered to offer euthanasia, through the proposed *Assisted Dying for the Terminally Ill* Bill (2004), to patients suffering unbearable terminal illness is likely to be opposed by Muslim clinicians; Muslims are of course not alone in this opposition:

> *The right to be spared avoidable pain is beyond debate — as is the right to say yes or no to some treatments... but once that has mutated into the right to expect assistance in dying, the responsibility of others is involved, as is the whole question of what society is saying about life and its possible meaning. Legislation ignores these issues to its cost.*
> Archbishop Rowen Williams (*The Times*, 20 January 2005: 21)

Cleanliness of body and mind

Notions of cleanliness are wide-ranging and will therefore impact extensively on day-to-day life. Thus, even when answering the call of nature, one is encouraged to be cognisant of the direction of the Kaaba (the Primordial House of worship in Mecca), signifying the direction of prayer, and if possible avoid facing it or indeed turning one's back towards it. After relieving themselves, many will use water to cleanse themselves and so water jugs or increasingly bidets are a common item in Muslim households or in public places in Muslim countries. Any cleansing of private parts is done with the left hand; the right hand is in contrast used for eating and handling/reading religious scriptures.

The ritual washing of exposed parts (wudu) before the five daily canonical prayers ensures physical cleanliness and furthermore, since this is also considered symbolically to wash away the excesses that the eyes, ears, nose, mouth or limbs may have committed, this also spiritually prepares the worshipper for his or her impending meeting with God.

Gender roles

Muslim women are often stereotyped in the West as being downtrodden and enslaved to their men-folk. However, according to the Qur'an: 'Women are the twin-halves of men' (Qur'an 2:228, 9:71, 16:89, 33:35) and 'equal and free partners to them' (Qur'an 30:21). Amongst Muslims, role demarcation is not considered sexist or discriminatory, but rather a reflection of a complementary and synergistic relationship (Gatrad and Sheikh, 2002) on which the family unit can be securely built and its integrity maintained (Dhami and Sheikh, 2000). A man is expected to go out and earn a living to support the family, whereas a woman's domain is primarily the maintaining of the house and the all-important role of nurturing children: both are complementary and essential, with neither having any greater inherent merit than the other. Of late, however, there has been a blurring of these roles as a result of acculturation. This process will, as has been the case in the West in general, contribute to the eroding of family values; the increases in promiscuity among Muslims and the rapidly increasing demise of the extended family unit are prime examples of this process. In spite of these worrying trends, there is still, relatively speaking, a strong family unit in most Muslim and indeed South-Asian households. Palliative care, which should begin from the time of breaking bad news, should therefore be delivered in a way that acknowledges and works with such considerations.

A further issue that is of relevance here is that of respecting modesty and, where possible, respecting sensitivities about being cared for by someone of the same sex. The dress code for Muslims should be such that it does not attract the attention of the opposite sex. There is therefore a reluctance on the part of some male and female patients of exposing their body parts before clinicians of the opposite, or increasingly of the same, sex. However, it should not be assumed that all Muslims subscribe to such mores and therefore polite enquiry, rather than simply assuming, is to be encouraged.

Conclusions

Islam is a global worldview and one that continues to expand wherever it has taken root. It is above all a faith that seeks to ensure the spread of peace and harmony and through doing so allows all individuals, irrespective of gender, colour or creed, to realise their God-given potential. Although certain contemporary developments may seem to suggest otherwise, for the vast majority of people, it remains a profound source of meaning, inspiration and hope. Occasionally, Muslim culture is at variance with the teachings of Islam. All that most Muslim patients ask for is an understanding of and respect for themselves and their religion by those who do not share it.

References

Al-Qaradawi Y (1985) *The Lawful and the Prohibited in Islam*. American Trust Publications, Indianapolis

---

Key points of *Chapter 3*

- 'Islam' in Arabic means 'peace and submission to divine decree'.
- Muslims follow the religion of Islam.
- There are over fifty countries with predominantly Muslim populations. Globally, numbers are estimated at 1.2 billion.
- Muslims are monotheists (they believe in a single god) and believe in a chain of guides from God who have been periodically sent as role models. Muhammad is but the last in this chain of prophethood.
- The Qur'an is the holy book for Muslims and this, together with the prophetic example, the Sunnah, forms the backbone of sacred law.
- Ijtihad or scholastic deduction combines with these two to give sacred law its inherent dynamism and contemporary relevance.

Dhami S, Sheikh A (2000) The Muslim family: predicament and promise. *WJM* **173**: 352–6

Gatrad AR (1994) Muslim customs surrounding death, bereavement, postmortem examinations and organ transplantations. *BMJ* **309**: 521–3

Gatard AR, Sheikh A (2002) Palliative care for Muslims and issues before death. *Int J Pall Nurs* **8**: 526–31

Gatrad AR, Sheikh A (2005) Risk factors for HIV/AIDS in Muslim communities. *DHSC* **1**: 65–9

Grayling AG (2005) Right to die. *BMJ* **330**: 799

Greenhalgh T, Collard A, Begum N (2005) Narrative-based medicine. *Pract Diabetes* **22**: 125–9

Kaymar MH, Roya P (2001) Issues in Islamic biomedical ethics: a primer for paediatricians. *Paediatrics* **108**: 965–71

Maria O'Beirne (2004) *Religion in England and Wales: Findings from the Home Office Citizenship Survey*. Home Office, London

Office of National Statistics (ONS) Census 2001

Williams R (2005) Does a right to assist a death entail a responsibility on others to kill? *The Times* **20 Jan**: 21

Winter TJ (2000) The Muslim grand narrative. In: Sheikh A, Gatrad AR (eds) *Caring for Muslim Patients*. Radcliffe Medical Press, Oxford

CHAPTER 4

Palliative care for Muslims

Rashid Gatrad, Aziz Sheikh

Every soul shall have a taste of death: and only on the Day of Judgement shall you be paid your full recompense.
Qur'an 2:185

Muslims follow the religion of Islam which traces its origins to the same semitic soil that bore Judaism and Christianity. Its most profound tenet is a belief in monotheism (a single god), summarised in the Declaration of Faith: 'There is no deity save God, and Muhammad is the Messenger of God'. This is whispered almost universally by Muslims into the ear of their newborn or a dying loved one. The daily life and body of Muslim communities pivot around this statement. Life's very purpose, then, is to realise the divine — an aspiration that is achievable only through a conscious commitment to the teachings of Muslim sacred law.

In this chapter, we consider issues before and after death for practising Muslims of South Asian origin, ie. those from India, Pakistan and Bangladesh. Implicit in our approach is a recognition that factors other than religion, such as culture, are also important in shaping the practices of Muslim minority communities in the UK.

Through sharing our multidisciplinary understanding and experiences, we hope to stimulate discussion and debate regarding possible strategies to raise awareness of Muslim culture. Our aim is to help facilitate a change in practice that will bring about care that is truly patient-centred.

Roughly one-third (over 600 000) of Britain's estimated 1.6 million Muslims trace their origins to the Indian subcontinent — that is, India, Pakistan and Bangladesh, sometimes referred to as South-Asian countries. Sizeable numbers come also from Europe (Albania, Bosnia, Cyprus and Turkey); Arabia (Iran, Iraq and the Arabian Gulf); and parts of northern and central Africa (Anwar, 2000). As our appreciation of the relationship between religion, health and health care increases, it is becoming increasingly apparent that the 'end-of-life' issues represent a period during which understanding and sensitivity are particularly important (*Panel 4.1*).

Panel 4.1: Case study — a mother's remarks after her daughter died of leukaemia

- Doctors were too busy and nurses were vague.
- Nobody was telling us directly what was happening.
- They were talking jargon.
- Nursing staff were rude and insensitive in repeatedly sending us home; I only wanted to be with my daughter as much as possible before she died.

Death — the Muslim context

In most societies, death represents the last great taboo. The thought of taking our final breath is something many of us consciously ignore. This tendency notwithstanding, death rituals for Muslims form the final bond between the deceased and the bereaved. As Muslims believe in an afterlife and the Day of Judgement, death is seen as a transition from one phase of existence to the next (*Panel 4.2*).

Islam teaches that life on earth is an examination, the fruits of which will be reaped in the afterlife. Death is therefore to be accepted as part of the divine plan and is not a taboo subject. Muslims are often encouraged to talk about death and reflect on their own existence in its context.

Types of patient requiring palliative care

The most common reasons for Muslim children to require palliative care are neuromuscular disorders, rare metabolic and genetic disorders and, to a lesser extent, cancers such as leukaemia (personal communication: Erica Brown, Acorns Hospice, Birmingham, UK, 2002). The most common reasons for adult Muslims to require palliative care are cardiovascular disease and the complications of diabetes, rather than cancer (Firth, 2001). Mortality from these two conditions in those over sixty-five has been found to be 55% higher in people from Pakistan and Bangladesh than in white people (Balarajan and Raleigh, 1995). Not only will there be a larger population of South Asians over sixty-five in the coming years, but there will also be a need for palliative-

---

Panel 4.2: The stages of life in the Muslim world view

- Life before conception: this stage refers mainly to a pledge made by each soul before entering this world to worship none other than God. The innate ability to perceive truth is considered a manifestation of this original divine encounter.
- The Lower World: life on Earth.
- The Intermediate Realm: from the time one departs from Earth until Judgement Day.
- The Garden and Fire: the eternal abodes.

---

care services to be increased by the likely breakdown of the extended family structure. We may therefore have to re-examine policies and systems if we are to meet demand over the next decade.

For Muslims, care of the dying — a regular and essential responsibility of extended family life — has, historically at least, been managed at home. There exist numerous traditions of the Prophet Muhammad (may God's peace and blessings be upon him), extolling the virtues of caring for the ill and particularly those in the last days of their life on earth. The aims of such 'care' are to encourage and support the dying and to cement firmly their relationship with God and kin before the imminent meeting with God on Judgement Day. The final illness thus represents a crucial period when people will wish to be surrounded by family and close friends who can take on the challenging task of fostering spiritual growth at this most vulnerable time. Palliative care of Muslims therefore involves not only the immediate and extended family, but also the Muslim community at large. Many may see being nursed by strangers in an alien secular environment as anathema. It is therefore not surprising that there exist very few hospices in the Muslim world; indeed, the terms 'hospice' and 'to palliate' have no direct equivalent in many South-Asian languages.

It is worth remembering that Islam has specific rules and regulations regarding a person's 'last will and testament'. In Islamic law, all children should receive a proportion of the estate of the deceased and the wife or husband should be included as beneficiaries.

Disclosure

Despite the points above, when reflecting on the inevitability of death and preparing for it assiduously, our experience suggests that many families do not wish their dying relative to be informed of the prognosis. The holding of conflicting narratives is perhaps not uncommon in all people at moments of uncertainty. It is sometimes suggested by relatives that information on prognosis should be given to the immediate relative who may or may not wish for a disclosure to the patient — a clear breach of confidentiality unless express patient permission has been given to do so. This is in keeping with Firth's observation (2001) that various minority ethnic and faith groups, including Muslims, often prefer non-disclosure for fear of triggering 'loss of hope'.

However, our experience also suggests that most, even the young, are usually aware that they are dying, at times as a result of cues picked up from parents and staff. Patients and relatives may also maintain a 'mutual pretence' (Bluebond-Langner, 1978). The reluctance of relatives and health professionals to talk about issues of death and dying affects the way a family copes with grief. We suggest that an honest yet sensitive approach is adopted when discussing prognosis. Note, however, that optimism and hope are regarded as some of the fruits of faith.

The main languages spoken by South-Asian Muslims are Urdu, Punjabi, Gujarati and Sylethi. Many will also have some understanding of Hindi. The provision of adequately trained interpreters is, where relevant, of paramount importance in facilitating communication. A study by Spruyt (1999) showed that when Bangladeshi children were involved in interpretation during the care of a dying relative, this had a negative impact on their school attendance — some gave up school and other older sons gave up work to look after their ill relative. Relatives of the ill, particularly if young, may be reluctant to talk about the illness to others if the illness is genetic, as it may affect the marriage chances of other members of that family.

Home, hospice or hospital?

In general, research has shown that when children die at home, long-term outcome is better for parents (Lauer *et al*, 1989). Making death clinical and having it occur in a hospital setting are not in keeping with Islamic tradition. The dying will expect to be visited by friends and relatives who are encouraged to pray for their welfare in the life to come. It is considered a Sunnah (a practice of Prophet Muhammad, may God's peace and blessing be upon him) to visit the sick. This is a time when Muslims seek each other's forgiveness for excesses that may have been knowingly or inadvertently committed in the past. Members of the immediate family will often stay by the bedside reciting from the Qur'an hoping to imbue peace and serenity into the heart of the loved one.

Patients sometimes tell us that prayers at home focus the mind better and therefore may help alleviate 'spiritual pain' better than saying prayers in institutional settings, which are often considered alien. In the Indian subcontinent, dying patients often return home to die. Although there is a dearth of research into the preferred place of death, a study by Gardener (1998) confirmed that among Muslim Bangladeshis, home was considered a sacred place to die. Some may, however, wish to travel abroad during their last illness. This is generally for one of two reasons. First, relatives may want traditional healers (Hakims and Pirs) to be consulted to see if they can effect a cure. Second, there may be a desire for death to occur in a sacred location such as the 'blessed' city of Mecca that is home to the Kaaba or Medina, the 'Enlightened city of the Prophet'. Should travel be anticipated for such purposes, it is important that the prognosis is discussed realistically as the opportunity for travel may slip away. Although Muslim undertakers in east London estimate that 60–70% of Bangladeshi corpses are repatriated (Firth, 2001), in our experience it is adults rather than children that are sent abroad for burial.

Prayers and spirituality

For Muslims, the spiritual dimension of death is paramount, since death marks the separation of the real and the surreal. Spirituality for Muslims is concerned with the transcendental, inspirational and existential way of being in relationship with God. This spirituality is heightened as the individual confronts death (Dom, 1999). Thus, the provision of adequate space for performing prayers and of prayer artefacts would be greatly appreciated by the family and community.

Muslims are expected to pray five times daily from the age of ten years (see *Chapter 3*). These prayers have a pivotal role in the lives of Muslims and assume an even greater role in times of distress for the family. Before prayer, ablution is performed; bed-bound patients will need help in this regard. Muslims pray facing Mecca. A specially designed compass is available from mosques and Muslim bookshops to identify the direction of prayer accurately. Many visitors will also often perform their prayers during visits to the hospital. Ablution facilities for the relatives and also the provision of a jug/plastic bottle in the confines of the toilet is a small but symbolic act that is greatly appreciated by Muslim families.

Practical aspects of care

Islam views life as a 'sacred trust' from God. Thus, suicide and deliberate euthanasia are categorically forbidden (Sheikh, 1998), as expressed in the Qur'an, 5:32: 'Whosoever takes a human life — it is as if he has taken the life of whole mankind'. Conversely, undue suffering has no place in Islam and, if death is hastened in the process of giving adequate analgesia, then there is no objection. Prolongation of life by artificial means is disapproved of by Islam unless there is evidence that a reasonable quality of life would ensue (Rahman, 1987).

A Tawiz or black string with a pouch containing religious scriptures may be tied to the wrist or around the neck of the patient. During practical procedures on the patient, this should not be disturbed without the consent of the patient or relative.

It is important to notify relatives that if opioids are used to control pain, this may have a negative impact on cognitive ability and levels of consciousness (see *Chapter 12*). This is because it will be hoped by relatives that the final utterance of the dying will be a reaffirmation of his or her Shahadah, the declaration of faith (*Panel 4.3*) in Arabic. During this process, the patient is also

Panel 4.3: The Shahadah

The Prophet Muhammad (may God's peace and blessings be upon him) taught:

Encourage your dying ones to say the affirmation of faith. Whosoever's final words are the Shahadah, 'There is no deity but God and Muhammad is the messenger of God', will enter the garden.

encouraged to drink water from the Well of Zam Zam, a process called Sakrat. Each family member present may attempt to give a sip of water to the dying. It is clearly important that this water is not inadvertently discarded. It is brought from Mecca in Saudi Arabia and may also be applied to various parts of the body of the dying. The presence of healthcare professionals who are unaware of these rites of passage may inhibit the relatives from performing it.

Muslims believe that their fate is sealed from the time of birth. This may be the reason why some Muslim patients are reluctant to undergo treatment, believing that to do so would be to defy God's will (Boyle, 1998). But this represents an incorrect understanding of scripture: active fatalistic thinking, which is common to all religious traditions in which God is omniscient (all-knowing), is very different from passive fatalism, which implies that we have no autonomous responsibility. Islam is above all a religion of justice and mercy: God only holds us to account over that which we have some control. Besides, the Prophet's repeated exhortations that 'for every disease God has sent down a cure' and stressing of the importance of 'seeking cure' are self-evident proofs that such notions should be open to challenge if encountered.

Withdrawing treatment

Withdrawing treatment from any patient is difficult. However, it is often easier for Muslim doctors, who share a common heritage and a world view, to withdraw treatment from Muslim patients than for clinicians from outside the faith. In such circumstances, after making it clear to the relatives that the patient's interests are our foremost concern, we have found that it is often possible to make use of Islamic teachings in counselling relatives regarding the difficult decisions ahead. We remind relatives of the transient nature of our earthly sojourn in contrast to the abiding reality of the afterlife. The exact time of death is a matter of divine decree over which we as fellow human beings are only bystanders.

In these situations we show guarded confidence in our ability to deal with the medical and spiritual aspects of the terminal phase and discuss the possibilities of how the illness will take its course. In the care of children, we remind parents that children are born pure according to the teachings of Islam and those (relatives) who remain true to their religion and abide by the teachings of sacred law will join their children in paradise.

Most Muslim authorities will consider brainstem death as an acceptable sign of death. A minority, however, are of the opinion that the concept of brainstem death is not acceptable in Islam and therefore argue that death is the point at which the soul departs — ie. complete cessation of any sign of life.

Issues after death

Death rites

When any Muslim dies, the eyes and mouth should be closed, the limbs straightened and the face of the deceased turned toward Mecca. Nurses can carry out these actions if relatives are not present. Professionals should however ensure that they do not leave the patient with feet pointing towards Mecca, as this may distress relatives. Ideally, a person of the same sex should handle the body unless the deceased is pre-pubertal.

Attempts should be made to release the body as soon as possible. There is a religious requirement to bury the deceased as quickly as possible. Burial within three to four hours of death would be normal in many Muslim countries for reasons that are both pragmatic and spiritual. Storage facilities are scarce and decay would set in quickly owing to the high temperatures in these countries. Rapid release of the body should help avoid unnecessary and prolonged distress to the bereaved family and friends. Muslim communities are closely knit and from our own personal experiences, more than 200–300 people visiting the home of the deceased would not be unusual. Thus, the longer the body remains unburied, the greater the burden on the family. In addition, many close relatives will not eat until burial, as a sign of respect. There is also the wish to allow the deceased to move on to his or her permanent abode: loved ones will of course be hoping that this is the Abode of Peace.

Washing and shrouding

It may take up to an hour for the body to be washed and draped in three pieces of simple white cloth. Usually, two people are needed for this procedure, which is carried out by Muslim members of the same sex as the deceased. The washing and shrouding of the body is usually carried out at a mosque. However, more and more hospitals are providing this facility for both sexes in a designated place in the mortuary. This practice, particularly for females, has, for example, been greatly appreciated by Walsall's Muslim community and we hope that such examples of best practice will be emulated in other regions and countries.

Post-mortems

The thought of post-mortems can create feelings of anxiety in the dying and their relatives. As Muslims are buried as soon after death as possible, problems arise if death is at a weekend or a post-mortem is planned. If a post-mortem is essential, this should be sensitively explained to the family. If it is not necessary, then it should be made clear that the family has a choice. The following scripture explains why post mortems are not allowed, unless the law of the country demands it: 'The breaking of a bone of the dead is equal in sin to doing that whilst he was alive' (al-Asqalami, 1996, quoting the Qur'an).

   Because of the psychological/emotional 'pain' often associated with post-mortems, the use of magnetic resonance imaging (MRI) scans instead of post-mortem examinations (Bisset, 1998) should be encouraged.

Organ transplantation

There is a verse in the Qur'an (5:32) cited by Yurdakok (2001), which is in support of organ transplantation: 'Whosoever gives life to a soul shall be as though he has given life to mankind'. Many Muslim scholars, particularly from the Arab world, agree that organs can be received both from Muslims and those of other traditions, based on the principle that the needs of the living supersede those of the dead (Baubaker, 2000). A person familiar with Muslim anxieties should be present at discussions regarding transplants so that concerns can be addressed accurately and sensitively.

Some other Islamic scholars from India and Pakistan, however, believe that the body is a 'trust' and therefore no one has the right to donate any part of it. The argument in favour of acceptance has not been helped by the illegal 'selling' of organs, as trafficking is forbidden by Islam. An important Fatwa (edict) from the UK-based Muslim Law (Shariah) Council in 1995 was strongly supportive of Muslims donating organs, and deserves wider circulation and debate (Anon, 1996). It is our opinion that this ruling will have widespread appeal, particularly among second- and third-generation Muslims who are educated in the UK.

Burials

In the unlikely circumstance of a Muslim dying with no relative or friend present, the elders of the Muslim community of that town will usually arrange for the ritual washing and the burial at their own expense. Muslims are always buried — never cremated. Often, members of the funeral committee collect the death certificate and make the necessary arrangements and leave the immediate family to receive visitors and grieve. When palliative care has taken place in the home, arrangements should ideally be made with the GP to ensure that in his or her absence a deputy is aware of the impending death. This may help to reduce some of the anxiety regarding an anticipated wait for burial. Some mosques have their own cold-storage fridges, but bodies are embalmed if burial is planned abroad. This custom is considered inappropriate and is now also declining owing to the expense involved.

Male community members follow the procession to the graveyard where a special prayer is offered and the deceased is laid to rest facing Mecca. To conform with UK practice, a wooden casket is provided by the mosque, this despite Islamic teachings stating that Muslims should bury their dead wrapped only in a white cloth. Some local authorities in the UK do now allow burial without a casket and have made provision for the issue of a 'disposal certificate' and burials at weekends. There does not appear to be a good reason for not acceding to the wishes of the Muslim community for the body to be buried without a casket, apart from this being different from accepted custom of the host nation. Muslim women will typically not attend burials (Gatrad, 1994).

Bereavement

Walker (1999) states that 'bereavement is the objective state of having lost someone, that grief is the emotion that accompanies bereavement and that mourning is the behaviour that social groups expect following bereavement' (see *Chapter 14*). Mourning is usually for a period of three days during which the mood is sad and yet reflective, with the positive aspects of the deceased being expounded. The inevitable sense of loss that occurs at the time of death is tempered by the belief that any separation is temporary, as Muslims believe in life after death. This sense of loss need not be a completely negative experience, as it represents an occasion to reflect on social and spiritual relationships, and indeed on the purpose of life itself.

Sabr is an Arabic word meaning 'unconditional contentment with the divine decree'. It is believed to represent one of the highest spiritual stations human beings can reach. Relatives and community members will encourage the family to practice and develop such 'contentment' in the 'hours of grief.' When the loss is of a child, the family will be reminded that children are pure and innocent and therefore assured of paradise (Tarazi, 1995).

The extended family networks of many Muslims provide support during illness and after death. The custom of talking through their experiences helps the bereaved feel less lonely and gives them the opportunity and the space to begin to heal. Muslims often have an explanation for a person's illness and death. The feeling of guilt, which is sometimes part of the bereavement process, is incorporated into the grieving process. This is dealt with openly rather than stoically, as often happens in the cultures of the West. Women may at times become animated in their expression of grief. Being present at the moment of death of a loved one can help the grieving process. An example of this can be seen in one Muslim mother's gratitude for being telephoned during the palliative care of her son (*Panel 4.4*).

Panel 4.4: Final moments

'I was rung up to say that Tahir was very ill. We rushed to be with him. He tried to smile, I squeezed his hand — he died. I will always be thankful for that call'.

The development of a Muslim bereavement service in east London alluded to by Firth (2001) could be emulated in other parts of the UK. Palliative-care services could also consider the appointment of Muslim 'chaplains'. Such professionals are able to offer emotional, psychological and spiritual support at this difficult time (see *Chapter 13*).

Effects of death on children

Children are often encouraged to visit the dying and male children may also attend funerals. It is important that children understand that it is not the dead body that goes to heaven, but the soul that 'flies' to be with God. The concept of the soul is, however, difficult for many to grasp. One explanation that may be given is that the patient was so ill that only God could make him or her better and that he or she will remain with God, and that we all meet at God's House when we die.

Strategies for change

The Acorns Children's Hospice in Birmingham, UK, is a prime example of how theory can be put into practice by understanding, in depth, the palliative-care needs of South Asians (see *Chapter 10*). Here, 30% of the 202 children registered were of South-Asian origin (Notta, 1998) and the large majority of these were Muslims. Familiarity with cultural diversity is therefore important in successfully delivering palliative care. A 'triangle' of health care exists, consisting of the client with his or her beliefs; the health professional with his or her beliefs; and the resources available to allow interaction between the two.

The principles of the four-step approach suggested by Kittler and Sucher (1990) (*Panel 4.5*) has great potential in the teaching and training of both nurses and doctors. Boyle (1998) suggests the use of a trans-cultural assessment model (Giger and Davidhizar, 1995) to help heathcare professionals become familiar with a client's culture. We would agree with this approach and give an adapted

---

Panel 4.5: Kittler and Sucher's model (1990)

- examine personal culture
- familiarise client culture
- identify adaptations made by the client
- modify client teaching based on data from earlier steps.

***Panel 4.6:* A transcultural assessment model**

- Explore professional caregiver's own personal culture.
- Become familiar with the patient's culture; issues include:
  - ❖ *communication*, ie. language, verbal and non-verbal cues
  - ❖ *space*, eg. for relatives to visit and pray if they wish
  - ❖ *social organisation*, such as family hierarchy
  - ❖ *time*, eg. how time is organised in relation to work and social aspects of life and timekeeping
  - ❖ *environmental factors*, eg. food, presence of religious artefacts
  - ❖ *biological variations*, eg. genetic variation in susceptibility to disease.
- Identify adaptations already made by the client, eg. may now be using toilet paper instead of water for toileting.
- Modification of emphasis in teaching, eg. targeting one of the parents or an elder family member to obtain accurate information and deliver education, eg. in home care.

Adapted from Giger and Davidhizar (1995).

version of the model in *Panel 4.6.*

Mandatory ethnic monitoring of routine healthcare service use, which began in the UK in 1995, should provide a more accurate record of those requiring palliative care. Data obtained from this should help improve palliative services. These services should involve not only the community leaders, but also the client group. Inclusion of religion in the data, as in the national census, may be a further step in refining services for ethnic-minority groups.

GPs are often the gatekeepers to palliative-care services. They, and other healthcare professionals, should be fully informed and educated about services that may be of particular value to certain cultural groups. For example, some families may find the Marie Curie night-sitting service of value, as, in our experience, many Muslims are night workers. This service provides respite for the family with a nurse staying the night with the patient in his or her home.

Helping families obtain appropriate financial help may also be very useful. This is particularly important because the carer may give up their job to look after the ill relative. A more culturally aware palliative-care service could theoretically be achieved by recruiting more nurses of South-Asian origin. However, nursing as a profession is often considered by Muslims to compromise values of modesty through dress code and handling people from the opposite sex. As a result, many parents in the UK will discourage their daughters from entering this profession. These barriers can of course be overcome.

Conclusions

Hospices conjure up visions of secular or Christian organisations. There is thus a need to ensure that all communities are aware of hospices and their role in providing palliative care for patients, irrespective of their religious beliefs. The lives of many Muslims, like most other South Asians, have a very strong religious basis. This means that cultural adaptations facilitating acceptance in the host culture may be slow. Although culture is dynamic, religious issues, particularly those surrounding birth and death, are likely to change more slowly.

Respect for the religion and culture of all faiths is important if health professionals are to deliver care that is truly patient-centred. For practising Muslims, the experience of death and dying represents a key time in the faith of the patient, their family and the community. In addition to offering understanding and respect, there are a number of practical measures that healthcare professionals can take to help Muslims at this time.

Key points of *Chapter 4*

- Learning and understanding some words in the language of the family is much appreciated by the families and helps create a bond. A simple Arabic greeting of 'Assalamu Alaikum' goes a long way in breaking barriers and creating trust.
- It would be helpful if hospitals/hospices provided:
  ❖ 'space' for relatives to visit in numbers and pray if necessary
  ❖ prayer artefacts in the form of mats, beads, incense sticks and a special compass for the direction of prayer towards Mecca.
- All religious books, such as the Qur'an, should be treated with the utmost respect by being kept on a separate shelf and only handled when covered with a clean piece of cloth/scarf. Audiotapes of the Qur'an should be made available if necessary.
- Advice from the Muslim 'chaplain' attached to the hospital should be sought in setting up appropriate palliative services.
- Nurses of the same sex as the patient should be involved with care and handling of the body.
- After death, the face of any Muslim, young or old, should be turned towards Mecca (south east from the UK). The feet of the deceased should *not* be allowed to face Mecca.
- Relatives should be notified of death immediately, as burial should take place within hours and the death certificate should be issued promptly.
- A post-mortem should only be requested if absolutely necessary.
- A bereavement officer/Muslim chaplain who can communicate in the appropriate language should be available.

Changes in the culture of South-Asian Muslims, such as the breakdown in the extended family, are likely to lead to an increased use of palliative-care services. There is therefore an increasing need for culturally sensitive services. We hope that our explanations of Muslim faith and culture will serve as a small step towards improved understanding between different cultures. Such improvements can only occur when health workers interact with the dying and the family in a spirit of compassion and understanding that allows them to feel accepted and valued. We healthcare professionals are capable of this great kindness — a kindness towards human life, which is a gift from God.

References

al-Asqalani AIH (1996) *Bulugh al-maram.* Dar-us-salam Publications, Riyadh

Anon (1996) The Muslim Law (Shariah) Council and organ transplants. *Accid Emerg Nurs* **4**: 73–5

Anwar M (2000) Muslims in Britain: Demographic and Socio-economic Position. In: Sheikh A, Gatrad AR (eds) *Caring for Muslim Patients.* Radcliffe Medical Press, Oxford

Balarajan R, Raleigh VS (1995) *Ethnicity and Health in England.* NHS Ethnic Unit. HMSO, London

Baubaker D (2000) Xenogreffe et bioetique Islamique. *Pathol Biol* **48**: 454–5

Bisset R (1998) Magnetic resonance imaging may be an alternative to necropsy. *BMJ* **317**: 145

Bluebond-Langner M (1978) Mutual pretence: cause and consequence. In: *The Private Worlds of Dying Children.* Princeton University Press, Princeton

Boyle DM (1998) The cultural context of dying from cancer. *Int J Palliat Nurs* **4**(2): 70–83

Dom H (1999) Spiritual care, need and pain, recognition and response. *Eur J Palliat Care* **6**(3): 87–90

Firth S (2001) *Wider Horizons.* National Council for Hospice and Specialist Palliative Care Services, London

Gardener K (1998) Death, burial and bereavement amongst Bengali Muslims. *J Ethn Migr Stud* **24**(3): 507–21

Gatrad AR (1994) The Muslim in the hospital, school and the community. Unpublished PhD thesis. University of Wolverhampton, Wolverhampton

Giger JN, Davidhizar RE (1995) *Transcultural Nursing: Assessment of Intervention.* 2nd edn. Mosby, St Louis

Kittler P, Sucher C (1990) Diet counselling in a multicultural society. *Diabetes Educ* **16**: 127–31

Lauer ME, Mulhern RK, Schell MJ, Camitta BM (1989) Long-term follow-up of parental adjustment following a child's death at home or hospital. *Cancer* **63**: 988–94

Notta H, Warr B (1998) Achieving accessible and appropriate services. In: Oliviere D, Hargreaves R, Munro B (eds) *Good Practices in Palliative Care*. Ashgate Publishing, Aldershot, Hants

Rahman F (1987) *Health and Medicine in the Islamic Tradition*. Crossroad, New York

Sheikh A (1998) Death and dying: a Muslim perspective. *J Roy Soc Med* **91**: 138–40

Spruyt O (1999) Community-based palliative care for Bangladeshi patients in east London: accounts of bereaved carers. *Palliat Med* **13**: 119–29

Tarazi N (1995) *The Child in Islam*. ATP, Indiana

Walker T (1999) *On Bereavement*. Open University Press, Buckinghamshire

Yurdakok M (2001) Paediatric ethics in the Holy Quran. *Arch Dis Child* **85**: 79–81

CHAPTER 5

The Hindu grand narrative

Shirley Firth

At the hour of death, when a man leaves his body, he must depart with his consciousness absorbed in Me.
Bhagavad Gita 8.5

The term 'Hindu' comes from a Persian-Arabic term for dwellers near the River Indus in the Punjab. Hinduism does not have an institutional framework, or demand adherence to particular doctrines, but is an 'umbrella' or 'family' of beliefs and practices. Each region in India has its own tradition and dialects. The concept of being a Hindu in India, a predominantly Hindu country, is considerably different from that in Britain. Hindus' sense of identity depends not only on their history, family, caste background and religious affiliation, but also on a complex of religious beliefs and attitudes.

Hinduism has a stratified social and ethical system, undergirded by the concepts of Karma and Dharma (below). Of particular importance is the concept of a good death — a prepared and conscious death, willingly faced in the belief that it is a transition to another life.

This chapter explores key Hindu concepts and provides some background in order that healthcare professionals in Britain can increase their awareness of the immense variations in language, caste system, religious practices, traditions and attitudes to disclosure and withdrawal of treatment. Some of these areas are revisited and expanded in the next chapter by Gatrad *et al* in the context of practical palliative care for Hindus.

Basic terms

Hinduism is sometimes termed Varnashramadharma. Each person is born into a Varna or a particular class, each of which is subdivided into occupation-based castes or Jatis, although today these have changed greatly. The four Varnas (classes) are:

- Brahmins (priests)
- Kshatriyas (warriors and kings)
- Vaishyas (merchants and traders)
- Shudras (peasants, labourers).

Historically, only the first three had access to Sanskrit, a language through which the ancient texts were transmitted. Men in these three Varnas were given a sacred thread at puberty, signifying their birth into adult life, and were hence known as 'twice-born'. Shudras (peasants) were regarded as 'clean' or 'unclean' (untouchable) depending on whether or not they were forced to deal with human waste and dead animals. Today, they are called Dalits, with active programmes of education and advancement.

Each class and caste has its own Dharma, which means righteousness, morality, or virtuous conduct, at personal, family, caste and universal levels:

> *... all the activities of the individual are fundamentally religious, and there is no aspect of life which can be divorced from Dharma.*
>
> Basham (1977: 244)

Dharma is therefore an ethical code of behaviour which relates to an idea of an underlying order and harmony in the universe, affecting human relationships, attitudes to health, wholeness and, ultimately, life and death.

There are ideally four stages of a life-cycle on earth called Ashramas:

- Brahmacharya — a student
- Grhasthya — a householder
- Vanasprastha (when grandsons have appeared) — a forest dweller
- Sannyasi — an ascetic.

This model is still socially and psychologically important to Hindus. For example, many elderly men and women 'withdraw into the forest', metaphorically speaking, when they in fact retreat into their homes, detaching themselves from material and emotional concerns and preparing for death through prayer, scripture reading and meditation. This may be the wish of the terminally ill.

Another important Hindu concept is Karma, the causal law in which all moral or immoral acts and thoughts have consequences in the next life. Good Karma leads to a good rebirth or liberation from the cycle of birth and death (samsara); bad Karma leads to a bad rebirth. Suffering can be explained in terms of past Karma.

Dharma includes ideas and rules about pollution relevant to each caste.

Dharma is particularly important in the context of death and bereavement. It is maintained by observing strict religious and caste rules regarding, for example, food (usually vegetarian) and ablutions following bodily functions and prior to prayer. Death is extremely polluting and, after a death, the family are bound by rules governing the 'purity' of its members during the mourning period, influencing what food can be offered to others, and restrictions about temple and domestic worship.

Most Hindus worship one or more divinities, regarded as manifestations of the one underlying reality, Brahman. Brahman is manifested as Brahma, the creator; Vishnu, the preserver; and Shiva, the destroyer. In practice, most worshippers are devoted to Shiva or his consort (Shakti, or female energy, appearing as Kali, Durga, Tara, Meenakshi or Mataji [Mother]); or Vishnu, who appears as a series of incarnations or avatars, to save mankind in times of need. The most popular of these Avatars are Krishna, with his consort Radha; and Rama, with his consort Sita. An ill Hindu may have one or more images of these deities around him or her. Even if a Hindu does not believe in any of these deities and classes himself as an atheist, he may still follow his Dharma.

Traditionally, for the twice-born, there are three paths to salvation: the way of devotion; the way of action; and the way of knowledge.

- *The way of devotion*: a Hindu may devote himself or herself to Rama, Krishna or Shiva, often within a sect founded or led by a particular teacher or Guru. This tradition is called Bhakti marga or yoga, the path of devotion, and decrees that the virtuous, with the grace of God, will go to heaven and obtain liberation from Samsara, the cycle of birth and death. The Bhagavad Gita is a favourite text for many Bhaktas.
- *The way of action*: a second group is made up of non-sectarian Hindus who describe themselves as Sanatana Dharm ('orthodox' Hindus) in the keeping of Brahmin priests, focusing on ritual action and possibly devotion to several deities. This tradition is sometimes described as Karma yoga, the way of action, the second path to salvation. This leads to a good rebirth.
- *The way of knowledge*: this third group, Jñana (gyan, in Hindi) yoga, believes in the way of mystical knowledge or enlightenment. In an important group of Hindu texts, the *Upanishads*, man's soul is identified with the Ultimate Reality, Brahman. Liberation from the cycle of birth and rebirth can be obtained through austerity, world-rejection and meditation, leading to mystical realisation of unity with Brahman in this life, and absorption into Brahman in the next (Moksha).

Hindus in Britain

After the Second World War, men — mainly agriculturists, craftsmen and Brahmins (class of priests) from rural areas or small towns — came to work in industrial areas of the UK, followed by relatives and then their families in a process of chain migration. They lived in clusters near each other, speaking the same language and maintaining connections with India by sending money back and arranging marriages.

In the 1960s, a new wave of middle-class Hindus arrived from East Africa as a result of 'Africanisation' policies there. Unlike earlier migrations, these 'twice migrants' came in familial, caste and sectarian groups (Barot, 1987; Clarke *et al*, 1990). Many had lost everything they owned in Africa, and struggled to establish new lives and occupations because their professional qualifications were not accepted in the UK. They began meeting in each other's homes to sing Bhajans (hymns) and pray, forming cultural associations that eventually led to the opening of local temples for religious and community use. The groups from Africa often observe different festivals compared with those directly from India, although there is often some syncretism (blending of traditions). Many temples have developed a Western style of Sunday 'service', to which members of different communities may come, although they are often dominated by certain groups, such as Gujaratis or Punjabis.

According to the 2001 UK census (http://www.statistics.gov.uk/census2001/census), there are currently over 558,000 Hindus in the UK, many of whom were born in this country. About 70% of the Hindu population is ethnically Gujarati, 15% Punjabi and the remainder are mainly from Uttar Pradesh and Bengal, with smaller numbers from Maharashtra and southern India. People from each region have their own tradition and dialect, and therefore caste groupings in different British cities vary considerably.

Sampradaya (sects) in Britain

Most Hindus in the UK belong to a Bhakti sect (Sampradaya), connected to the teaching of a guru or gurus.

- Most Gujaratis follow Swami Narayan, a nineteenth-century reformer considered to have been an avatar of Vishnu. They have constructed a huge temple in Neasden (north London). Others belong to Pushtimarga, worshipping the infant Krishna. The International Society of Krishna

Consciousness (ISKCON, Hare Krishna), also devoted to Krishna, was founded in the West by Swami Bhaktivedanta Prabhupada, and has many Western followers. Sathya Sai Baba, regarded by many as an incarnation of Shiva, is a living guru in southern India, with thousands of Western as well as Indian devotees.

■ Many Punjabis belong to Arya Samaj, a nineteenth-century reform movement rejecting image worship and 'orthodox' rituals in favour of ancient Vedic ones (based on the ancient texts, the Vedas), the most important of which is Havan, the Vedic fire ritual.

Despite the above differences, there are common presuppositions about the nature of family life and care of the dying. In India, the extended or joint family enables elderly people to be cared for at home, which is where one should die when there is no hope of a cure. Many hospitals in India make provision for the family to stay with the patients, prepare the correct (usually vegetarian) food and undertake their physical and emotional care. Patients may go home to die. With a higher mortality rate, and because people often die at home, death is familiar, even to children, who are not excluded from the death bed.

In the UK, where the extended family system is fragmenting with social mobility and lack of space, the sick and the elderly cannot always be cared for at home. Most deaths occur in hospital, and medical personnel may have little understanding of a Hindu's traditions, religious or social needs, with different assumptions about dying and death. For example, crowds around the bed of a dying person to say goodbye and perform religious rituals, and emotional responses to a death, can be disruptive on busy wards. Yet failure to be with a dying person, from both personal and religious perspectives, can be catastrophic for relatives, leading to long-term guilt and anxiety. For many Hindus, the rituals (or the failure thereof) actually affect the progress of the soul (below).

After the death of a loved one, relatives have to face the 'professionalisation' of death and bureaucracy. Changes in the timing of funerals and problems of cremation upset traditional mourning patterns. In India, cremation is usually within a few hours of death, after which mourning rituals begin. In the UK, there is often a delay of a week before crematorium 'space' is given. The brevity of the cremation service may shift the focus from concern for the departing soul to the comfort of the mourners. Specialist priests for the post-death rites may not be available. All this can lead to a feeling of loss of control.

Beliefs about life and death

Most Hindus believe that there is a soul (Atman) in all living beings, which transmigrates from one life form to another in a cycle of birth and death

(Samsara). In the Bhagavad Gita, Krishna, the supreme lord, creator of the universe, describes the indestructible nature of the Atman:

There was never a time when I did not exist, nor you, nor any of these kings. Nor is there any future in which we shall cease to be. Just as the dweller in this body passes through childhood, youth and old age, so at death he merely passes into another kind of body...

Bhagavad Gita 2. 12-13, 17

All action should be selfless, without any thought for its fruits (karma), motivated only by the love of God. Those who love God, and think of Him at the time of death, will come straight to Him:

Then he will be united with Me... Whatever a man remembers at the last, when he is leaving the body, will be realised by him in the hereafter; because that will be what his mind has most constantly dwelt on, during this life.

Bhagavad Gita 8.5

For many Hindus, this passage is the key to a good death (infra vide), focusing only on God and not on the world one is leaving behind, as that hinders one's progress in the next life.

A religious scripture called the *Garuda Purana* (c. 800–1000 CE) has had a major influence on popular beliefs today. It is often read during the mourning period, but may be rejected as too depressing. It describes the soul's post-mortem journey for a year through numerous temporary hells, and prescribes the rituals the relatives have to perform to release the ghost of the deceased and create a new ethereal body for its disembodied soul. These are now condensed into the twelve days (a symbolic year) following death, culminating in a powerful ritual, the Sapindikarana, in which the deceased becomes an ancestor and the mourners return to normal life. Until then, the relatives are in severe ritual impurity and live austerely.

In addition to temporary heavens, where the virtuous are rewarded prior to rebirth, some devotees believe that the virtuous will remain permanently in heaven with their God. For example, Swaminarayan followers, who practise Bhakti yoga, will reside in His abode, Akshardham.

Good and bad deaths

For Hindus, a good death is in old age, at the right astrological time, and in the right place, at home if it cannot be on the banks of the Ganges. It should be prepared for throughout life, and entered into consciously and willingly (Firth, 1997). All affairs should be set in order, marriages arranged for daughters or granddaughters, conflicts resolved, and gifts of money and land made.

It is important to say goodbye to relatives and friends, and the last words are highly treasured, becoming part of the way tradition is passed on (*Panel 5.1*).

For a good death, a Brahmin priest may facilitate an act of penance. To ensure that the dying person focuses on God, devotional hymns are sung or religious words such as 'Ram Ram' or 'Om' are chanted. Just before death, the person is laid on the floor, Mother Earth, with the head to the north, which enables the soul to leave freely. Death on a bed shows lack of care. Ganges water and a Tulsi (basil) leaf are placed in the mouth, to purify the body and cleanse the soul of sins (Firth, 1997).

Signs of a good death are a 'shining forehead' and a peaceful expression, with eyes and mouth slightly open, indicating the soul has departed. In holy individuals, the soul leaves from the top of the head. Bad deaths are violent, premature and uncontrolled, in the wrong place and at the wrong time, signified by vomit, faeces, urine and an unpleasant expression (Parry, 1982; Firth, 1997). For example, a Gujarati woman, who died in the lavatory with a horrible expression on her face, was considered to have had a particularly bad death.

Providing the right rituals to 'see the soul on its way' is a profoundly sacred debt for a son. Without these rituals, the soul may not move on, haunting the relatives or causing bad luck, nightmares, illness and infertility. One Gujarati family was forbidden to give a tiny sip of Ganges water to a dying aunt. 'The doctors said that she would live a little longer, but there was no point, she was dying anyway. They switched off the machine, and they said they mustn't give her anything that would give her a shock and kill her straight away…' (Firth, 1997: 117–8). In consequence, her nephew and his wife believed that her restless soul was responsible for their infertility, and that her unsatisfied soul would affect the family for seven generations unless they performed a long and expensive ritual, in India, for all the relatives.

Panel 5.1: A good death for a Hindu

My mother was like a saint and she died in just five minutes. She was 103 years-old and she could put thread into needle. She walked without a stick. She asked for a bed on the floor… Then my sister's son came. He said, 'What's happening, Bibi?' She said, 'O thank God you came. Come and give me [a light] on my hand [to show me the way to God]'. My sister started crying and she said, 'Don't cry. Your tears will make a river for me to cross. I'm going to God. Let me go first. Don't stop my way'. He did everything, [then] she said, 'Put my head in your lap. I want to go to God'.

Firth (1997: 58).

Disclosure

As in many other cultures, there is a tradition of non-disclosure for many Hindu families (Gordon and Paci, 1997; Ng *et al*, 2000). This creates a tension between autonomy, which ensures knowing the prognosis in order to prepare for a 'good end', and being protected from this knowledge by relatives in case the person gives up hope and dies prematurely. Furthermore, modern medicine provides hope, however unrealistic, that a cure is possible. Sudhir Kakar, a psychiatrist, argues that the death of an individual, particularly a parent, ruptures the extended family system: '[This] not only brings a sense of insecurity in a worldly social sense, it also means the loss of "significant others" who guarantee the sense of sameness and affirm the inner continuity of the self' (Kakar, 1987: 121).

Although there is a strong Hindu tradition of being prepared for death, not all deaths are those of the elderly who have fulfilled their life's goals. This can create problems of disclosure and withdrawal of care. In India, the patient may be taken home or to a bhavan (home for the dying), which implicitly discloses to the patient that death is imminent.

The difficulty of open disclosure is illustrated by an example of a Gujarati man, Suresh, and his son, Ramesh, in England (*Panel 5.2*).

Panel 5.2: The difficulty of disclosure — Suresh and Ramesh

A Hindu GP warned Ramesh that his father was terminally ill with prostate cancer and, later, tuberculosis. Ramesh did not want his father told his prognosis. Unfortunately, the doctors reassured Ramesh that Suresh would recover, and his prognosis was never discussed openly. However, he was clearly aware that he was dying, giving his books away, talking about dying, and obtaining a gold chain for his granddaughter's marriage, but colluding with his son's silence. When Suresh died unexpectedly in his son's absence, Ramesh was racked with guilt because he had not been present to give his father the last rites or say goodbye.

(Firth, 1997).

Willed death and voluntary euthanasia

In a 'good', conscious and willed death, the body is relinquished voluntarily. There has long been a tradition of voluntary death and, indeed, of religious suicide in some Hindu traditions. Such a self-willed death was 'linked to a specific purpose: to obtain freedom (heaven or liberation) thorough an act of omnipotence, involving the sacrifice of the self' (Young, 1996: 83). Terminally ill individuals may fast to achieve spiritual purification, promote detachment, and ensure that there are no post-mortem signs of a bad death — eg. faeces, vomit or urine (Firth, 1997). Medication may be accepted in order to die with a clear and unclouded mind, viewing pain as a way of expurgating sin (Firth, 2001) and suffering as a 'purifying and cleansing' process. This can cause problems for Western-qualified professionals whose training makes them want to maintain life and relieve suffering.

A more difficult issue is the withdrawal of treatment from those unable to give consent, especially if the family resists. In the earlier example of the aunt in the Gujurati family, it was accepted that death was imminent because of her stage of life. However, when a three-year-old Punjabi child had been knocked down by a car, it took three days for the family to understand the concept of brain death and give permission for withdrawal of life support.

There is a distinction between the willed death of a spiritually advanced person, and someone in great pain wishing to end an intolerable life. Hindus perceive suicide for selfish reasons as morally wrong, and such a death cannot normally have the all-important post-mortem rites (shraddha), although some Hindu lawgivers have made exceptions (Kane, 1974). Some recent authorities argue that only God can take life, and humans should not do so because of the karmic effect on the next life (Crawford, 1995). Subramuniyaswami, a Hindu scholar, states that 'a lethal injection severs the astral "silver cord" connecting the astral body to the physical. Those involved then take on the remaining karmas of the patient' (Crawford, 1995: 109). Crawford, however, suggests that according to Ayurvedic medicine, it should be morally possible for a terminally ill person who is suffering greatly to choose the time of his or her death, otherwise he may lose 'the equanimity he so cherishes for his final moments of life. Euthanasia ensures a merciful death because he can leave this life with consciousness unclouded by the stupor of drugs, and without fear that some bad karmas will plunge him back into mortal existence' (Crawford, 1995: 111). This would be more difficult for people who are not spiritual adepts, but the arguments below might be adapted for such cases.

Hindu ethics discourages involuntary euthanasia because, from a Hindu perspective, it contradicts the principles of justice and autonomy and can lead to abuse. However, the primary concern is the relief of suffering. Mohandas Gandhi (1869–1948) — more commonly known as 'Mahatma' ('great-souled') Gandhi — advocated Ahimsa (non-violence), which is 'uttermost selflessness', refraining from any harmful act. Yet it was necessary to destroy some life in order to live at all, and sometimes one has to take life to protect others. Gandhi could not abide the thought of allowing a rabid dog to die a painful death. He hoped there would be better remedies for human beings in a similar situation:

Should my child be attacked with rabies and there was no helpful remedy to relieve his agony, I should consider it my duty to take his life. Fatalism has its limits. We leave things to fate after exhausting all remedies. One of the remedies and the final one to relieve the agony of a tortured child is to take his life.

Cited in Young (1996: 116)

There are, therefore, different levels of Ahimsa. Evil may be eclipsed by a compassionate act performed selflessly because ultimately it is the intention that counts. This might be applied, for example, to a severely disabled baby with a poor prognosis. Crawford comments:

Karma does not give us the right to keep such people alive and in pain when all they want is a peaceful death. Their Karma is our Dharma. We have a duty to our fellow human beings. If they are suffering because of some sin, it is not less a sin to let them suffer. Mahatma Gandhi had said, 'God comes to a hungry man in the form of a slice of bread! In what form does God come to a person begging to die?'

Crawford (1995: 116)

There is thus not a single moral position on the issue of involuntary euthanasia and there remains a long-standing tradition of voluntary suicide in certain carefully defined circumstances.

Conclusions

The complexity of Hindu belief and practice makes it important not to generalise about Hindu patients at the end of life and to avoid a 'shopping-list' approach to their needs. Hindu beliefs and attitudes depend on education, class and religious tradition. Professional carers need to discover the individual patient's and family's particular religious position to enable him or her to have a good death with their help. Health professionals may already be deeply and actively involved in discussions about prognosis, and home care should be provided if requested. It is important to acknowledge the long-term importance of allowing the right deathbed rituals to take place, recognising the tension between allowing for patient autonomy and disclosure and the need for the family to make decisions on behalf of the patient. The Hindu good death provides a valuable model for how death can be approached positively and without apprehension in the context of a supportive family and religious beliefs.

Key points of *Chapter 5*

- Hindus have many different traditions, languages, migration histories, and ranges of social status and education.
- Most UK Hindus belong to devotional sects, which influence their behaviour and attitudes to suffering and death.
- Most Hindus believe in an eternal soul, which is reborn until it becomes pure enough to reach heaven or be liberated.
- A good death is prepared, conscious, with the mind focused on God. Relatives should help the dying to achieve a good death.
- There may be tension between disclosure, autonomy and the right of relatives to take charge.
- Voluntary euthanasia may be justified in some circumstances.

References

Barot R (1987) Caste and sect in the Swaminarayan movement. In: Burghart R (ed) *Hinduism in Great Britain: the Perpetuation of Religion in an Alien Cultural Milieu*. Tavistock, London

Basham A (1977) Hinduism. In: Zaehner RC (ed) *The Concise Encyclopedia of Living Faiths*. Open University Press and Hutchinson, London

Bhagavad Gita (1963) *The Song of God*. Trans. Prabhavananda, Swami and Isherwood C. Mentor Books, New York

Clark C, Peach C, Vertovec S (eds) (1990) *South Asians Overseas: Migration and Ethnicity*. Cambridge University Press, Cambridge

Crawford S (1995) *Dilemmas of Life and Death: Hindu Ethics in North American Context*. State University of New York Press, USA

Firth S (1997) *Dying, Death and Bereavement in a British Hindu Community*. Peeters, Leuven

Firth S (2001) *Wider Horizons: Care of the Dying in a Multicultural Society*. National Council for Hospice and Palliative Care Services (NCHSPCS), London

Gordon D, Paci E (1997) Disclosure practices and cultural narratives: understanding concealment and silence around cancer in Tuscany, Italy. *Soc Sci Med* **44**: 1433–52

Garuda Purana (1979) Part II. Part III. Trans. Board of Scholars. Motilal Banarsidass, Delhi

Kakar S (1987) *The Inner World: a Psychoanalytic Study of Childhood and Society in India*. Oxford University Press, Delhi

Kane PD (1974) *History of Dharmashastra*. Vol IV. Bhandarkar Oriental Institute, Poona

Ng NF, Shumacker A, Goh G (2000) Autonomy for whom?: a perspective from the Orient. *Palliat Med* **14**: 163–4

Parry J (1982) Sacrificial death and the necrophagous ascetic. In: Block M, Parry J (eds) *Death and the Regeneration of Life*. Cambridge University Press, Cambridge

UK Census (2001) Available from http://www.statistics.gov.uk/census2001/census (accessed August, 2005)

Young K (1996) Euthanasia: traditional Hindu views and the contemporary debate. In: Coward H, Lipner J, Young K. *Hindu Ethics: Purity, Abortion, and Euthanasia*. State University of New York, Albany

CHAPTER 6

Palliative care for Hindus

Rashid Gatrad, Pamela P Choudhury,
Erica Brown, Aziz Sheikh

There was never a time when I did not exist, nor you, nor any of these kings.
Nor is there any future in which we shall cease to be. Just as the dweller in this
body passes through childhood, youth and old age, so at death he merely passes
into another kind of body.
   Bhagavad Gita

Health professionals are increasingly encouraged to focus on the idea of a 'good death'. In addition to physical and psychological support, this should include supporting religious perspectives to provide truly holistic care. This article highlights issues before and after death that are potentially relevant to healthcare professionals caring for terminally ill Hindu patients in the UK. In providing such care, they should be aware of the process of acculturation, leading to erosion of traditional support networks. Such networks have hitherto been crucial buffers during times of distress and grief. Healthcare professionals should aim to develop cultural competence, based on improved understanding rather than simply an increase in cultural knowledge (Webb and Sergison, 2003).

The Hindu community worldwide

The majority of the UK's 558,000 Hindus originate from the Indian subcontinent. There is also a sizeable community from East Africa (Kenya, Tanzania, Uganda and Malawi). This latter group are unusual as they have twice migrated in their recent history, first from India to east Africa and then to the UK. Hindus have also migrated to Malaysia, Fiji and the West Indies. In the UK, areas such as Harrow (north-west London), Leicester and Brent (north

---

Panel 6.1:The Om symbol

Om is the aksara or imperishable syllable.
Om is the universe and this is the exposition of Om.
The past, the present and the future — all that is, all that will be, is Om...
Likewise all else that may exist beyond the bounds of time, that too is Om.

(Radhakrishnan, 2001).

London) have significant Hindu communities, making up 14–19% of the local population (Office for National Statistics [ONS], 2003). As with most religions, differences in emphasis and interpretation have, over generations, resulted in diverse practices, which are to an extent dependent on language, region, caste affiliations and sectarian considerations.

An overview of Hinduism

Hinduism is a religion of thousands of gods and goddesses and it is generally accepted that these are all different manifestations of the one God. Families may choose to 'adopt' a particular deity and have a shrine at home with a statue or picture of the chosen deity. In the UK, the majority of Hindus are Vishnuvites, meaning they follow Vishnu (the Preserver: see *Chapter 5*) (Neuberger, 1994). The most important Hindu symbol is the Om (*Panel 6.1*).

The Bhagavad Gita (Radhakrishnan, 2001) is one of the four main scriptures important to Hindus. These texts were originally written in Sanskrit, a language in which relatively few Hindus are now literate. Many Hindus will therefore have learnt religious principles by the ancient traditional system of Katha, the passing of knowledge from one generation to the next by word of mouth.

Issues before death

The Hindu concept of death

In *Chapter 5*, Shirley Firth alludes to the Hindu scriptures, which teach that there are four stages in the earthly sojourn (*Panel 6.2*) (Neuberger, 1994).

Panel 6.2: The Hindu concept of death

- Bramacharya – period of education
- Garhasthya – working in the world
- Vanaspatha – the retreat for the loosening of ties and worldly attachment
- Pravrajya – the awaiting of freedom through death.

Stages three and four are perhaps of most interest to those involved in providing palliative care (Neuberger, 1994). In the third stage, the individual, although beginning to become aloof from this world, still keeps in touch with it by imparting to it his or her worldly wisdom. In the fourth stage, those relationships are gradually severed so that the spirit can be released to unite with the Supreme Being. The individual is not supposed to allow life to come to an abrupt end, but should achieve this reunification gracefully. If the latter occurs, it should bring considerable comfort to the dying Hindu and his or her family (Neuberger, 1994).

Belief in Karma is the most important of all Hindu religious doctrines. Karma is defined as 'deeds' (Chan *et al*, 2003) that refer to actions in the present and previous life. Hindus believe that, according to the law of Karma, the process of birth and rebirth of a soul depends on the deeds of that person in their previous life. Thus, after death, the 'soul' is transferred into a new body. Samsara — that is, the process of birth, death and rebirth — continues until one's Karma is such that a new plane of existence, Moksha (liberation), is reached. Hindus believe that this is a state of divine reincarnation, when a soul is at one with God. Karma will therefore often have a strong influence on attitudes towards illness and death.

The caste system

Although not officially recognised and less visible in modern-day India than in the past, the caste system still has a strong hold on Hindu families, and its impact often extends to families that have migrated. Closely linked with reincarnation, the caste system is based on the belief that everyone is born into a particular caste, depending on one's past deeds in a former life. Caste often determines a person's occupation in India, although less so now than previously.

Types of patients requiring palliative care

Hospice and specialist palliative-care services traditionally focus on patients with cancer (Smaje and Field, 1997; Tebbit, 2000). Cancer in the UK is more common in those over fifty-five years-old. However, because of the younger demographic profile of many migrant communities, its incidence is, at present, lower among South Asians than among the white majority population (Rawaf and Bahl, 1998). Other conditions, such as vascular diseases and diabetes mellitus, for which there is much less specialist palliative-care service provision, are more common causes of death among Hindus (Balarajan and Bulusu, 1990). Palliative care for people with non-neoplastic terminal disorders is often a challenge because the pattern of deterioration may be less predictable and it is often more difficult to assess prognosis reliably when compared with cancer patients (Steinhauser *et al*, 2001).

Hindu practices may influence some disease patterns. For example, a strict vegetarian who has a diet high in dairy fat may be more prone to coronary heart disease (Nazroo, 1997). Similarly, a vegetarian diet is said to be a factor in the low rates of breast cancer in Asian women (Hoare, 1998). It cannot, however, be assumed that second- and third-generation migrants who develop cancer will have the same specialist palliative-care needs as the first-generation migrants or the indigenous population in view of the process of acculturation.

Care of the dying

For Hindus, care of the dying is typically seen as a family responsibility. Terminally ill patients will thus (at least at present) seldom ask for respite or nursing care from specialist palliative-care providers.

Death, a profoundly spiritual time, is typically associated with a number of rituals. It is important that every attempt is made to ensure that family members have the opportunity to be present to undertake these rituals to help ensure a 'good death.' All relevant health professionals should ensure that they are aware of the principles of a good death for all denominations.

Nursing staff may only allow limited visiting by the extended family if relatives are deemed to be noisy, intrusive and present in too great a number. It is, however, believed by Hindus that it is important to hear and acknowledge the last words of a dying relative as these may be of spiritual significance. Such words could indicate a good or a bad death, providing the family with some insight into the next 'journey' of the departed soul.

Disclosure

In common with many Chinese people (Tong, 1994), many Hindus believe that discussion of death may make it more likely to occur. Thus, by discussing death, one is almost 'willing' death on the dying relative. In the authors' experience, many Hindu families will also be reluctant for their dying loved one to be informed of their clinical condition, resulting in a 'conspiracy of silence' in order to protect their dying one. Such practices can bring families into conflict with health professionals.

Elderly Hindus in the UK will typically speak Gujarati, Punjabi, Bengali or Hindi. The services of adequately trained interpreters are therefore important in any discussions. Studies on care given to patients in the last year of life confirm that poor communication with patients and their relatives is common (Addington-Hall *et al*, 1998; Fakhoury, 1998).

Home, hospice or hospital?

It is widely recognised that many South Asians prefer to die at home (O'Neill, 1994). Research has shown that the next most preferred place of death is the hospital, which is perhaps unexpected, given that notions of a clinical death are not in keeping with the Hindu faith (Choudhury, 1999). Some specialist palliative-care units have traditionally had a Christian image and Hindu patients may be reluctant to be admitted to such units (Karim *et al*, 2000) at a time when spiritual care is of major importance. However, anecdotally, they and their relatives often readily accept admissions to hospitals named after a saint.

Another factor in the preference for home deaths is the wish to avoid bad luck. Units where dying patients are being looked after may be perceived by some as being tainted, with the risk that such units could bring bad luck upon families. Hence, there may be reluctance to attend centres specifically associated with cancer. This reluctance to accept inpatient specialist palliative care has also been recorded on the Indian subcontinent (Burn, 1997). Thus, the under-use of inpatient specialist palliative care occurring both in the UK and the Indian subcontinent may be a matter of cultural stigma (attached to the word 'hospice') in addition to inadequate and inaccessible facilities.

For many Hindu patients (in common with other South Asians), the administration of an intravenous fluid is often regarded as a defining procedure, indicating that a patient is seriously unwell. Withdrawal of food and water is unlikely to be considered acceptable as both are believed to be central to a good death. Relatives may turn to hospital units where palliative care does not include such withdrawal.

Rashid Gatrad, Pamela P Choudhury, Erica Brown, Aziz Sheikh

In the Indian subcontinent, patients and families are often of a different social class to doctors. Patients may therefore experience difficulty in communicating their fears and needs to healthcare professionals. As a result, they may find it easier to seek advice from a traditional healer, who plays a major role in Indian society, especially in rural areas where about 80% of India's population lives. Anecdotally, migrants to Western countries do seek such advice rather than formal health care. Some Hindus may choose to return to their homeland in order to die there. Even though such deaths often occur without freely available opiates or specialist palliative-care services, they are still regarded as good deaths (Joranson *et al*, 2002).

Panel 6.3: Best practice for Hindu patients before death

- *Icons* — the dying Hindu may wish to have a small statue or picture of the family god to be brought in and placed at the bedside. Such icons need to be treated with respect by hospital/hospice staff.
- *Bathing* — bathing or washing must occur with fresh running water. The Western custom of bathing in a tub of water is regarded as unclean.
- *Holy water* — Hindus consider the Ganges a holy river and its water sacred. The family may place a few drops of this water and a tulsi (basil leaf, also regarded as sacred) into the mouth of the dying patient.
- *Oil lamps* — families may choose to light small oil lamps and burn incense in the patient's room. If relatives are prevented from performing these sacred rights, it is believed that the soul of the dying patient will be impeded on its next journey.
- *Prayer* — patients may need Mala (prayer beads). Puja (prayer mats) are traditionally offered at sunrise and Hindus have a strict ritual of defecation, bathing, the wearing of clean clothes, and fasting before prayers. This enables them to communicate with God in a purer form.
- *Modesty* — in common with many South-Asian faiths, modesty is of utmost importance to Hindus. Help with dressing or bathing by a healthcare professional of the opposite sex is often considered unacceptable. Similar problems can occur in the reluctance to discuss issues regarding bowels and micturition.
- *Diet* — 'diet-Hindus' consider the cow to be sacred and beef is therefore not eaten. Indeed, some devout Hindus will be vegetarian. Such individuals often stipulate that their food be prepared in a kitchen that has not had beef (or, for the very strict vegetarian, any meat, fish or eggs) prepared in it. As this is usually not possible in hospitals or indeed specialist palliative-care units, consideration should be given to the possibility of relatives bringing in food from outside.

Prayers, pain and medication

For the dying, the requirements may simply be to move the bed into a quiet room where the patient may wish to pray and meditate. Hindus commonly combine prayer, meditation and exercise in a disciplined way.

It is believed that when a Hindu experiences pain, suffering or distress, it may be as a result of his or her own sinful acts or evil deeds, not only in this life but also in past lives. Our experiences suggest that there has often been a reluctance by dying Hindu patients to report pain. This may be because of the belief in Karma; Hindu scriptures extol that pain must be endured, just as pleasure is to be welcomed. Death is a natural phenomenon and therefore need not be feared. Many people believe that, through meditation, one can ignore, forget or detach oneself from physical pain. By becoming at one with God, it is believed that one can divert one's mind from such physical problems. To achieve such a higher state of mind, a clear consciousness is required and Hindu patients may therefore be reluctant to use strong analgesics, particularly opioids. Health professionals may find the practice of voluntarily enduring pain difficult to accept.

Withdrawal of treatment, and death

Vomiting and incontinence of any sort are often regarded as signs of a bad death. As Hindus regard death as a process of Karma, the withdrawal of futile treatments is generally acceptable. Most Hindus will have accepted their illness in a stoical and fatalistic way. Therefore, many patients may choose to prepare their bodies for death by fasting, as this will ensure that they are 'pure' at the most auspicious of times in their lives. In this way, the approximate timing of death may be estimated by the patient who hopes to die with full consciousness and without the fear of bad Karma (Firth, 2005). In some holy places in India, such as Varanasi, fasting before death is common and accepted.

As patients approach death, the family will chant 'Ram Ram' or 'Om' and recite from the Bhagavad Gita (Radhakrishnan, 2001). Religious words or Mantra are whispered into the ears of the dying patient. A thread with a religious significance may be tied around the wrist or neck by a priest. The patient may chose to lie on the floor in order to be close to Mother Earth when he or she dies. *Panel 6.3* summarises best practice for Hindu patients before death.

> ### Panel 6.4: Best practice for Hindus after death
>
> - After death the body should be placed on the floor with the head facing north.
> - If relatives are not present, they should be notified immediately.
> - The death certificate should be issued promptly together with appropriate paperwork to ensure cremation.
> - A post-mortem should be requested only if absolutely necessary.
> - People of the same sex should handle the body after death. Non-faith members may handle the body.
> - A bereavement officer who can communicate in the appropriate language should be available.

Issues after death

After death, the body is traditionally placed on the floor (*Panel 6.4*). People of the same gender should handle the body, although it does not necessarily have to be members of the same faith. Water from the river Ganges is used to purify the body, with a few drops being placed into the mouth of the dead person. In addition, a Tulsi (basil) leaf together with a small fragment of gold (to symbolise the paying of the ferry man crossing the river of death) are placed in the mouth. The facial expression of the deceased is considered important: if it is serene, with the mouth and eyes slightly open, this is believed to indicate a good death.

No jewellery, sacred threads or other religious insignia should be removed from the body. The precise ritual around preparation of the body depends on caste and family traditions. A local Brahmin (priest) may be called to oversee preparations. A deceased man would be dressed in normal clothing and a woman in a Sari or Shalwar kameez. A widow is typically dressed in white. The body may be placed in a coffin and taken home for final viewing. Here, the family members may wish to circumambulate the coffin to bid farewell. There will be recitations from the Bhagavad Gita and oil and incense will be burned (Radhakrishnan, 2001).

Post-mortems

There is no specific Hindu prohibition of post-mortems (Schott and Henley, 1996). However, discussions relating to these, as in all cases, need to be handled sensitively, as many believe that cremation of an incomplete body will result in the soul not being reborn but forever suspended in a 'state of animation'. This in turn could bring bad Karma to the family.

Cremation

It is customary not to bury Hindus, but rather to purify them by fire through cremation. The only exception to this rule is children, who are buried. It is believed that children have unformed personalities and, therefore, do not need to undergo the ritual of purification. As cremation should occur as quickly as possible after death; every effort should be made to issue death certificates and the necessary paperwork for cremation promptly.

Male relatives will accompany the body on the journey to the crematorium. Traditionally, female members are not permitted to attend the ceremony. It is the duty of the eldest son to activate the fire in the crematorium and perform this final ritual. Considerable distress occurs in families who have no sons or close male relatives. Exceptions have been made when daughters or female relatives are allowed to take on this important duty. However, this is often at the behest of the overseeing Brahmin. After cremation, the ashes, together with any bony fragments, are scattered into the Ganges or in other holy places. In the UK, the ashes are often saved and, when convenient, taken to India. An acceptable alternative to many families is to sprinkle the ashes into a local river (such as the Thames for communities in and around London).

Bereavement

The quality of palliative care has an impact on bereavement and mourning (Koffman and Higginson, 2001). Hindus who have witnessed what they perceive as their relative's bad death may be very anxious about the ghost of the deceased (Firth, 2001). Attention to spiritual belief in palliative care may therefore provide an existential framework in which grief is resolved more readily (Walsh *et al*, 2002).

After death, there follows a formal mourning period of between ten and sixteen days. Bereaved families are regarded as tainted after a death and, therefore, friends and relatives will not eat or drink at their house. During the mourning period, relatives eat simple food and dress without adornment. Some may not cut their hair or nails and this extends to men not shaving. Days will be spent reading the Bhagavad Gita and other religious texts. On the twelfth day, the soul of the deceased is said to be recreated. On the same day, nails and hair may be cut and men may shave their beards and traditionally some will shave their heads too. In practice, in the UK, these ceremonies tend to occur on the day of death. After the formal mourning period, a Shraddha is held. This is akin to a wake, when family and friends are invited to the bereaved family's house.

Effects on the family

CancerLink, an organisation that specialises in networking self-help groups, has identified that the belief — commonly held by health professionals — that minority ethnic families prefer to rely on their own resources and do not need help from outside agencies can result in a lack of support for carers (Faull, 2003). One study (Choudhury, 1999) has shown that the uptake of bereavement services offered by specialist palliative care units is so poor that informal bereavement support is essential. The extended family members are often able to do this if they themselves have experienced bereavement and are able to share their mutual experiences. Often the overwhelming theme in the bereavement process is that the deceased will have moved onto a better life.

Young Hindus in the UK will have little or no experience of death rituals and yet will be expected to lead the rituals after death. They often find themselves 'lost' at a time when they too are grieving. If they are expected to return to the Indian subcontinent to attend ceremonies, the sense of alienation and bewilderment is compounded. Bereavement services in the UK may therefore need to respond to both the young and the old. A good model of such an innovation is that of the City and East London Bereavement Counselling Service, UK, where Muslims are trained to act as bereavement counsellors for their community (Firth, 2001).

Strategies for change

Since the publication of the National Council of Hospice and Specialist Palliative Care Services document, *Opening Doors* (Hill and Penso, 1995), various strategies have been implemented to make specialist palliative-care services more accessible to minority ethnic groups in the UK. These have had varying degrees of success. One of the reasons why such services may not be accessed by minority ethnic groups is that patients are not aware of them because the information, when provided, is not in the appropriate language (Iqbal *et al*, 1995). To address this problem, the South Asian Palliative Care Arts Awareness Project (SAPCAA) was established in 2001 in Birmingham through the New Opportunities Fund, a distributor of money raised by the National Lottery. In *Chapter 9*, Faull and Thakker discuss how such a project can help improve understanding of and access to palliative care through, for example, the use of a Hindi drama called 'Humara Safar' ('Our Journey').

Although most Hindus tend to register with an Asian GP, it cannot be assumed that the doctor will have an understanding of the patient's religion or culture. Therefore, organised systems of information should be available to all healthcare professionals, including GPs who are often the gatekeepers to specialist palliative services.

Over recent years, in the UK, there has been a breakdown of the extended family network (Sheikh and Gatrad, 2003) — a phenomenon not exclusive to Asian families — which has implications that are twofold. First, the breakdown of this essential support structure often leaves elderly Hindus more vulnerable; strategies to aid communication through trained interpreters and advocacy therefore need to be in place. Second, as the burden of care often falls onto a few individuals, more and more families in the future may request respite care.

The current models of hospice care have hitherto not been culturally accepted by many first-generation Asians (Hill and Penso, 1995). As future generations develop higher cancer rates and social changes occur, they may be more receptive to existing models of care. Certain aspects of specialist palliative care, which are already used and are culturally acceptable to Hindus, could be developed further — for example, domiciliary home care, day care and hospice at home. Unfortunately, most services in the UK are suffering from a decline in continuity of care as a result of restructuring of medical training and shift-working (Finlay, 2003). Even the out-of-hours nursing services are fragmented. If integrated care pathways are introduced in palliative care (Ellershaw *et al*, 1997), their audit should ensure that issues relating to care of ethnic minorities are addressed.

Conclusions

Culture and religion affect one's perception of health and illness. Times of distress, such as serious illness and bereavement, cause a community to lean towards their own culture. Attempting to alleviate all distress with a generic — that is, Western — palliative approach may not be appropriate.

Cultural competence is an evolving process that depends on self-reflection, self-awareness and acceptance of differences. It is based on improving understanding, as opposed to an increase in cultural knowledge (Webb and Sergison, 2003). With this philosophy in mind, we have attempted to address some of the key issues for Hindus relating to death and dying. We hope that this chapter will help those involved in the palliative care of Hindu patients increase their understanding of, and ability to meet, each individual's unique palliative-care needs.

> **Key points of *Chapter 6***
>
> - Hinduism is one of the world's oldest religions and traces its origins to the Indian subcontinent.
> - Hindus are now to be found throughout the world.
> - Underlying the often complex array of deities is a central belief in a Supreme Being.
> - Health professionals need to be aware of key rites of passage in the period preceding death that are, if not adequately addressed, believed to impact negatively on future cycles of birth and death.
> - Facilitating a prompt cremation can help the grieving process.

References

Addington-Hall JM, Walker L, Jones C, Karlsen S, McCarthy M (1998) A randomised controlled trial of postal versus interview administration of a questionnaire measuring satisfaction with the use of services received in the year before death. *J Epidimiol Community Health* **52**: 802–7

Balarajan R, Bulusu L (1990) Mortality among immigrants in England and Wales. In: Britton M (ed) *Mortality & Geography: a Review in the Mid-1980s*. HMSO, London

Burn G (1997) Palliative care in India. In: Clarke D, Hockley J, Ahmedzai S (eds) *New Themes in Palliative Care*. Open University Press, Buckinghamshire

Chan KP, Pickering M, Pai S, Sheikh A, Soloman A (2003) Doctors and their faith. *BMJ* **326**: S135–8

Choudhury PP (1999) A Comparison of the Uptake of Specialist Palliative Care Services by Asian and White Patients in Wolverhampton. MMedSci dissertation. University of Keele, Keele

Ellershaw J, Foster A, Murphy D, Sjea T, Overill S (1997) Developing an integrated care pathway for the dying patient. *Eur J Pall Care* **4**(6) 203–7

Fakhoury WKH (1998) Satisfaction with palliative care: what should we be aware of? *Int J Nurs Stud* **35**: 171–6

Faull C (2003) Cancer and palliative care. In: Kai J (ed) *Ethnicity, Health and Primary Care*. Oxford University Press, Oxford

Finlay I (2003) Dying with dignity. *Clin Med* **3**: 102–3

Firth S (2001) *Wider Horizons: Care of the Dying in a Multicultural Society.*

National Council for Hospice and Specialist Palliative Care Services (NCHSPCS), London

Firth S (2003) End of life — A Hindu view. *Lancet* **366**: 682–6

Hill D, Penso D (1995) *Opening Doors: Improving Access to Hospice and Specialist Palliative Care Services by Members of the Black and Ethnic Minority Communities.* NCHSPCS, London

Hoare T (1998) Breast cancer. In: Rawaf S, Bahl V (eds) *Assessing Health Needs of People from Minority Ethnic Groups.* Royal College of Physicians, London

Iqbal H, Field D, Parker H, Iqbal Z (1995) Palliative Care Services for ethnic groups in Leicester. *Int J Pall Nurs* **1**: 114–6

Joranson DE, Rajagopal MR, Gilson AM (2002) Improving access to opioid analgesics for palliative care in India. *J Pain Symptom Manage* **24**: 152–9

Karim K, Baily M, Tunna K (2000). Non-white ethnicity and the provision of specialist palliative care services: factors affecting doctors referral patterns. *Palliat Med* **14**: 471–8

Koffman J, Higginson IJ (2001) Accounts of carers' satisfaction with health care at the end of life: a comparison of first generation black Caribbean and white patients with advanced disease. *Palliat Med* **15**(4): 337–45

Nazroo JY (1997) *The Health of British Ethnic Minorities.* Policy Studies Institute, London

Neuberger J (1994) *Caring for Dying People of Different Faiths.* 2nd edn. Mosby, London

Office for National Statistics (ONS) (2003) www.statistics.gov.uk (accessed October 2005)

O'Neill J (1994) Are ethnic minorities neglected by palliative care providers? *J Cancer Care* **3**: 215–20

Radhakrishnan S (2001) The Bhagvad Gita. HarperCollins, India

Rawaf S, Bahl V (1998) *Assessing Health Needs of People from Minority Ethnic Groups.* Royal College of Physicians, London

Schott J, Henley A (1996) *Culture, Religion and Childbearing in a Multiracial Society.* Butterworth-Heinemann, London

Sheikh A, Gatrad AR (2003) Children and young families. In: Kai J (ed) *Ethnicity Health and Primary Care.* Oxford University Press, Oxford

Smaje C, Field D (1997) Absent minorities?: ethnicity and the use of palliative care services. In: *Death, Gender and Ethnicity.* Routledge, London

Steinhauser KE, Christakis NA, Clipp EC *et al* (2001) Preparing for the end of life: preferences of patients, families, physicians and other care providers. *J Pain Symptom Manage* **22**: 727–37

Tebbit P (1999) *Palliative Care 2000: Commissioning through Partnership.* NCHSPCS, London

Tong KI (1994) The Chinese palliative patient and the family in North America: a cultural perspective. *J Palliat Care* **10**: 26–8

Walsh K, King M, Jones L, Tookman A, Blizard R (2002) Spiritual beliefs may affect outcome of bereavement: prospective study. *BMJ* **324**: 1551–4

Webb E, Sergison M (2003) Evaluation of cultural competencies and antiracism training in child health. *Arch Dis Child* **88**: 291–4

CHAPTER 7

The Sikh grand narrative

Jagbir Jhutti-Johal, Sukhvinder S Johal

Truth is the highest of all things,
And higher still is truthful living.
  Guru Granth Sahib

Sikhism is one of the world's youngest religions. Its founding Guru or enlightener, Nanak, was born in 1469 CE ('Common Era', equivalent in years to AD) in Punjab, which literally means 'a land of five rivers', an area that resides across India and Pakistan. From a small movement of kindred spirits, Sikhism has now grown into a religion of about twenty million people (see www.sikhs.org.uk). In their short and turbulent history, the Sikh people have been key players in many of the major events of Indian history in the past 500 years, including the fall of the Moghul Empire; the rise of the Sikh Empire in Punjab under Ranjit Singh; and the rise and fall of the British Empire and the Indian independence struggle. Over the past century, Sikhs have migrated overseas in substantial numbers. As a result of this diaspora, Sikhs are to be found in several countries outside India, primarily in the UK, USA, Canada, East Africa and Malaysia.

Sikhism has its roots firmly embedded in Eastern philosophy. It shares many of its theological concepts — such as Samsara, the cycle of birth and rebirth; Karma, the law of action; and Moksha, liberation or salvation — with faiths such as Hinduism and Buddhism, although its interpretations of these concepts may be somewhat different. In common with many Semitic faiths, it is an ardently monotheistic tradition (worship of a single deity) that advocates the belief that God created the universe and everything that exists within it. God is thought to be beyond human comprehension and formless (Nirankar). Sikhs can accept that the central figures of other faiths, such as Krishna, Moses, Jesus and Muhammad, were messengers of God with a divine mission. However, they do not accept the authority of any of the scriptures from other religions. Sikhs also do not believe that God takes a human form and hence reject the idea of, for example, the divinity of Jesus Christ or the gods or Avatars of Hinduism.

The word Sikh is derived from the Sanskrit word 'Shishya', which means a 'disciple' or 'learner'. This embodies the mindset of Sikhs, who are on a continual quest towards the path to enlightenment. This enlightenment generally involves the guidance of the Guru, which now is manifested in the form of the Guru Granth Sahib, the holy book of the Sikhs. Some dimensions of Sikhism discussed in this chapter are explored further in *Chapter 8*, where the authors discuss practical aspects of Sikh palliative care.

A short history

The history of Sikhism is one of enlightened souls; spiritual reinvigoration; beautiful poetic literature; martyrdom; and struggle against persecution. Sikhs derive tremendous strength from their history. Guru Nanak was born during a relatively peaceful period in northern India following waves of invasions by Turks and Afghans as well as domestic anarchy. Despite this original peace, the years of war and toil had left an indelible mark on its people. The period was one of great uncertainty, ignorance and moral disintegration. Society was fragmented, not just by the rivalry of the two main religions, Hinduism and Islam, but also by the divisions within these religions. The caste system led to religious and racial segregation: the performing of perfunctory rituals in the name of God had permeated through society and superstitious practices were rife. For Guru Nanak, the world had entered a dark age in which most people had become disenfranchised from the path to salvation, and religion had lost its true purpose, the path of truth:

> *The times are like drawn knives, kings like butchers,*
> *Righteousness has fled on wings,*
> *The dark night of falsehood prevails,*
> *The moon of truth is nowhere visible.*

Guru Granth Sahib

Nanak's life coincided with a period of religious renaissance in Europe, Martin Luther (1483–1546) and John Calvin (1509–64) being among his contemporaries (Singh, 1999). He challenged current theologies and preached the message that the liberation of the soul was open to all, irrespective of race, sex, caste or religion. He may have drawn some inspiration from Sufism, a branch of Islam that emphasises spirituality and the Bhakti, or 'devotion to God' movement that had originated in southern India. However, he ultimately fashioned his own philosophy, elevating 'Truth' to the highest status and recognising God as one. In practical terms, Nanak convinced people that the Creator was immanent (present everywhere) and accessible to everyone; he also encouraged charitable works and selfless service and promoted the cause of women.

Before his death, Nanak appointed a successor, Angad, to continue his mission. In all, there were ten human Gurus, each of whom is accorded equal status. In fact, for many Sikhs, the Gurus are seen as the spirit of Nanak assuming ten forms and in the Guru Granth Sahib, subsequent Gurus are referred to as Nanak I, Nanak II, and so forth. Each Guru advanced the faith and added various facets to it. Angad collected Nanak's hymns into a book and added his own compositions. He also gave Sikhs a new script, Gurmukhi (from the mouth of the Guru), which gave the Sikhs a written language distinct from the written language of Hindus and Muslims, and thus fostered a sense of their being a separate people (Singh, 1977).

As the number of Sikhs began to grow, the third Guru, Amar Das, began the institutionalisation of the Sikh faith. He appointed territorial ministers, made the system of Langar, or Guru's free kitchen, an integral part of religion. He also introduced social reforms, such as the prohibition of Sati, the burning of widows on their husband's funeral pyres, allowed remarriage of widows, advocated monogamy, denounced the veiling of women, and appointed women preachers.

Ram Das, the fourth Guru, established a village, which was eventually to become the city of Amritsar, the spiritual and political capital of the Sikhs. The fifth Guru, Arjan, oversaw the construction of the holiest shrine in Sikhism, the Harimandir, now known as the Golden Temple. Arjan was a prolific writer and composed more hymns than any of his predecessors. His most important achievement was the compilation of the Granth Sahib, an authoritative collection of his work and the works of the first four Gurus. Also included were the works of Hindu and Muslim saints whose views echoed that of the Gurus. The Granth Sahib was installed at the Harimandir in 1604 CE. The Granth Sahib became the embodiment of Sikh thought and more than anything helped to catapult Sikh teachings to a wide audience. Arjan wrote of the Granth Sahib:

In this vessel, three things lie:
Truth, contentment, contemplation.
They contain the ambrosial Name,
By which we are all sustained.
They who eat, they who savour, they are liberated.
This thing must not be abandoned;
Ever and ever, keep it in your heart.

Guru Granth Sahib

The growing influence of Arjan brought him into conflict with the rulers of Punjab. Indeed, his presence may have been seen by the authorities as a threat to their power. The Mughal Emperor, Jehangir, had Arjan arrested and while in custody Arjan was put to death. He is seen by Sikhs as their first martyr and his death marked a turning point for the Sikh community, which now felt a real and physical threat to their principles and way of life. The sixth Guru, Hargobind, in reaction to this, added a militaristic dimension to the Sikh faith. He introduced the concept of the Guru not only having spiritual authority (Piri), but also assuming a temporal role (Miri), that is, of or relating to worldly matters. The period of Guruship among the seventh and eighth Gurus was generally one of peace and the continual spread of Sikh teachings. This peace was to be shattered during the tenure of the ninth Guru, Tegh Bahadur. He died defending the rights of others to practice their own faith. Like the fifth Guru, Tegh Bahadur was executed by the authorities. Tegh Bahadur composed many hymns, which were later added to the Granth Sahib by the tenth Guru.

The tenth Guru, Gobind Singh, was instrumental in creating the Khalsa (the fraternity of the 'pure') which instructed Sikhs to take Pahul (baptism) to create a community devoted to a life of prayer and service, as well as being prepared to fight injustice and defend the weak. He also introduced the outward symbols of Sikh identity worn by 'baptised' Sikhs, known as the five Ks (see *Chapter 8* for greater detail): Kara (steel bangle); Kirpan (small sword); Kesh (uncut hair); Kanga (comb); and Kshera (soldiers' short breeches). Further, to emphasise the equality of man and rejection of the caste system, all men who joined the Khalsa were to add the name Singh or 'lion' to their forename and all women were to add Kaur or 'princess'. However, today virtually all Sikhs, whether baptised or not, will use Singh or Kaur as a middle name. On the eve of his death, Guru Gobind Singh, decreed that no living Guru would follow him and that spiritual authority now rested with the Granth Sahib. This holy book was now to be the eternal Guru of the Sikhs.

With each Guru there was most definitely a shift in emphasis of the Sikh movement. This was in part a natural evolution of a religious movement and in part a response to the changing political and social circumstances. However, it is quite clear from the Guru Granth Sahib that the core spiritual or religious ideology did not change.

The Guru Granth Sahib

In terminal care, in our experience, the recitation of scriptures from this holy book is encouraged and widely practised, as the Guru Granth Sahib is the epitome of the spiritual teachings of Sikhism. It is the Sikhs' perpetual guide and contains the main doctrine of Sikhs concerning God, God's nature and attributes, and the means by which salvation may be attained (Field, 1914). Sikhs view it as the repository of God's word transmitted through His messengers, the Gurus. As Nanak stated,

I speak, O God, only when you inspire me to speak.

Guru Granth Sahib (p. 566)

Guru Granth Sahib is not written as a moral code or as a document recording history. The paucity of references within the Guru Granth Sahib describing contemporary historical events or moral dilemmas is an indication that the Gurus wished it to transcend these superficial issues and focus on the timeless and eternal Creator (*Panel 7.1*).

Indeed, many would argue that the Guru Granth Sahib is simply an attempt to explain the first line in it, Ek Onkar, meaning 'there is but one God'. Guru Granth Sahib is the main focus at all Sikh ceremonies, including birth, marriage and death. It is held in such high veneration that it is wrapped in a fine cloth and Sikhs will prostrate themselves before it when entering its presence. Its hymns are usually expressed musically. The Guru Granth Sahib is testament to a unique feature of Sikhism, that the word of the Guru (or God), Gurbani, is the key to salvation and not the Guru himself. The Guru is the instrument that God uses to spread His Word. Therefore, handling this book, and indeed all other religious books, should be with utmost humility and respect.

Panel 7.1: A description of the Guru Granth Sahib given by Pearl S. Buck, winner of the 1938 Nobel Prize for Literature (Buck, 1987)

Shri Guru Granth Sahib is a source book, an expression of man's loneliness, his aspiration, his longings, his cry to God and his hunger for communication with that being. I have studied the scriptures of other great religions, but I do not find elsewhere the same power of appeal to the heart and mind as I feel here in these volumes. They are compact in spite of their length, and are a revelation of the vast reach of the human heart varying from the most noble concept of God to the recognition and indeed the insistence upon the practical needs of the human body. There is something strangely modern about these scriptures and this puzzled me until I learnt that they are in fact comparatively modern, compiled as late as the sixteenth century, when explorers were beginning to discover the globe upon which we all live as a single entity divided only by arbitrary lines of our own making. Perhaps this sense of unity is a source of power I find in these volumes. They speak to persons of any religion or of none. They speak for the human heart and the searching mind.

Who is a Sikh?

Sikhs can essentially be divided into two main groups: the baptised and the non-baptised. The pahul ceremony (Amrit Sanskar) is undertaken when an individual fully comprehends the implications of such an act. Hence, it is rare for a prepubescent child to be baptised. There is no upper age limit to baptism and it is encouraged for both men and women. The ceremony takes place in the presence of the Guru Granth Sahib. The principles of the faith and other key instructions on how a baptised Sikh must live are imparted to the initiate. For example, these include devotion to God; service to mankind; fight against injustice; and defence of the weak. On acceptance of these instructions, Amrit (nectar of immortality) is prepared by pouring water and sugar pellets in a steel bowl and stirring the mixture with a double-edged dagger while selected verses from the Guru Granth Sahib and Dasam Granth (collected works attributed to the tenth Guru) are read aloud. Five handfuls of Amrit are drunk by the initiate and five handfuls are sprinkled over their hair and eyes. Further prayers are then offered followed by a random reading of a verse from the Guru Granth Sahib. If a person does not have a Sikh name, they take a new name at this time. The candidate is now formally admitted to the Khalsa community (Gatrad *et al*, 2005).

Baptised Sikhs (Amrit-dhari or Khalsa Sikhs) constitute an 'orthodoxy' within Sikhism. Non-baptised Sikhs (who form the majority in the UK) are either Kes-dhari Sikhs (keep their hair unshorn and wear the outward symbols of the Sikh faith, ie. the turban) or Mona Sikhs (retain an affiliation to the Khalsa, but remove the outward symbols of the faith) (Gatrad *et al*, 2005). All Sikhs will believe in the one eternal God, the ten Gurus and accept the Guru Granth Sahib as their eternal Guru.

The ultimate reality

The central statement of the Sikh faith about God is given in the opening lines of the Guru Granth Sahib. Composed by the first Guru, Nanak, these provide a succinct summary of the very essence of Sikh beliefs about God:

> *There is One Supreme Being*
> *Eternal Truth by Name*
> *Immanent in all beings*
> *Sustainer of all things*
> *Creator of all things*
> *Without fear*
> *Devoid of enmity*
> *Timeless in image*
> *Beyond birth and death*
> *Self-existent*
> *Made known by the grace of the Guru.*
>
> Guru Granth Sahib (p. 1)

The unity and oneness of God is a theme continually repeated throughout the Guru Granth Sahib. God is also described as formless, without gender and, in common with many religions, beyond human comprehension. God is the creator and the cause of creation. The essence of God is known as Naam and this pervades all creation. Sikhs believe that every soul is a divine spark of the eternal flame of the Creator and the ultimate aim is for each spark to obtain union with its divine source.

The human condition and spiritual liberation

The ultimate goal in Sikhism is to achieve Moksha (liberation) from the cycle of birth, death and rebirth and union with God (Sahaj). Birth can take the form of any one of 840,000 life-forms. The human form is seen as the only opportunity to break this cycle and fulfil one's destiny. Thus, human beings are thought to be blessed by having reason, wisdom and the potential for being aware of God. Guru Nanak preached the message that this liberation or salvation was open to all, irrespective of caste, creed or sex. However, the goal of liberation is not an easy one to achieve and ultimately depends upon God's grace.

The key obstacle to achieving liberation is Haumai. This is a very difficult word to translate into English, but can be interpreted as an inner egoistic self-centred being. All men and women are born with haumai, which is God-created, and it acts like a veil, obfuscating the presence and vision of the divine that pervades all around and within each person. According to the Gurus, haumai is the great disease of humanity (Singh, 1994). Haumai leads the mind and soul into delusion and worldly attachment.

The Guru Granth Sahib elucidates how liberation can be achieved and calls for a self-centred approach to be replaced by a God-centred approach to life. The aim is to achieve a new state of consciousness and realise God within. The most important concept is that of Naam Simran or 'meditation of the True Name'. Some Sikhs will use the technique of constantly repeating God's Name, but Naam Simran goes well beyond this. The mind must be wholly tuned to the essence of God so that the person becomes totally absorbed in Him. Now every thought and action has to be imbibed with God. Ultimately, this is done without any mental effort or any conscious awareness and the result is a person who dedicates his or her life to God and the service of others. Naam Simran is not something to be done alone or away from society and certainly does not advocate withdrawal from daily life. It should be accompanied by participation in the life of Sangat, the fellowship of believers (Cole and Sambhi, 1978), and as an active member of the community.

Nanak describes five realms or levels of spiritual experience as one traverses the path to union with God. The final level, the realm of Truth, leads to the realisation of the Truth and complete harmony with God. In contrast to many religious traditions, one does not have to wait for death to achieve this state of being. Liberation is available in this present life. Death only marks the final release.

The discipline of Naam Simran and the final goal of union with God is certainly not an easy one. Many Sikhs accept that they will not reach the realm of truth. However, for them, the goal is certainly one worth striving for and they recognise that sincere efforts can make it achievable.

Sikhism rejects asceticism, renunciation of worldly life, celibacy, or the separation from one's family or home to achieve union with God. Married life, Grihasta, is celebrated and encouraged.

Sikh practices

In a multicultural society where people of different faiths may look after a very ill Sikh patient and perhaps continue to interact with the family after death, the following section will, we hope, be of practical help. All religious movements, if they are to last, ultimately develop a set of rules and practices to give the message of their founders permanency and also to bond the disciples of that movement closer together. Sikhism is no different in this regard. Most of these practices date back to the time of the Gurus, but have been formalised in the last two centuries. They are a reinforcement of the teachings of the Gurus.

The central pillar of Sikhism is Naam Simran — a quest to connect with the Creator, which overrides all else. This should be coupled with a life dedicated to truth and service of others. Sikhism rejects the idea that fasting, bathing at religious sites, religious penances or pilgrimages have any spiritual merit:

If salvation can be achieved by bathing in water, then a frog is better off. He remains in water all the time.

Guru Granth Sahib (p. 484)

The daily routine of a Sikh dates back to a practice introduced by Guru Nanak. While every Sikh should attempt to keep God in his thoughts constantly throughout the day, there are three set prayers to aid meditation. First, he will rise at dawn and, after taking a bath, will meditate by reciting a selection of hymns composed by Guru Nanak and Guru Gobind Singh. Next, at sunset, he or she will recite the Rahiras (the Holy Path) and finally, before going to bed, will repeat a payer called Sohilla. While there are no ritual ablutions before prayer, bathing is seen as essential for personal hygiene and in helping to reinvigorate the mind and body for meditation. The daily prayers are performed by oneself, collectively as a family, or at the Gurdwara (Sikh place of worship).

The gurdwara, meaning 'doorway to the Guru', is the centre for all Sikh worship and it is where the Guru Granth Sahib is mounted. For Sikhs, the gurdwara represents a place for meditation and contemplation where one can be infused and energised by listening to the recitation of the Guru Granth Sahib. Inside the gurdwara, worshippers will approach the Guru Granth Sahib and genuflect (kneel) or prostrate themselves fully before it, before sitting down. This should not be confused with idol worship — this act is performed to accept the authority of the Guru Granth Sahib and its teachings. The general convention is to sit on the floor, but for the infirm or disabled, chairs or wheelchairs are permitted. Men and women usually sit on separate sides of the Guru Granth Sahib, which is in keeping with Indian cultural norms. There is no fixed day for worship, but in the West, congregations usually gather in large numbers on Sunday, reflecting the cultural context in which Sikhs live. Music and the singing of hymns are seen as integral to meditation and worship. Music is seen as a way of lifting hearts and minds and helping to ease one's attention towards God.

Sikhism has no priesthood or ordained ministers. Any baptised lay member of the congregation may lead the worship, male or female. In practice, many Gurdwaras, especially in the West, employ a Granthi ('reader'), usually male, whose responsibilities include reading the scriptures, performing ceremonies and the upkeep of the gurdwara. However, his role should not be confused with that of a priest; he does not have any special religious authority above that of an ordinary lay member, but will invariably be well-versed in the scriptures. Although some Granthis may undertake hospital visits, most Sikhs will seek the guidance of devout friends, relatives or other community members (particularly elders) in times of need.

In keeping with the principle of equality, the gurdwara is open to all people of any religion (or of none), nationality, caste, gender, and so forth. This openness is extended to the langar, the 'Guru's free kitchen', in which vegetarian food is prepared and served to the congregation. All partakers will sit together on the floor and eat — this is another expression of equality. The langar is an integral part of worship.

It is worth mentioning at this point that while the founders of Sikhism set out to establish a society based on equality and free of caste hierarchies, in practice, Sikh societies have absorbed some aspects of Hindu caste practices. Sikh villages in India are still divided in much the same way as Hindu villages (Bhachu, 1985), with different castes sitting on different rungs of the social ladder. These ideas also persist in the minds of Sikhs outside India, including in the UK. Traditionally, the Jats (agriculturists) have resided at the top of this caste hierarchy and form the majority of the Sikh population in India and the UK. They are followed by castes such as Ramgarhias (artisans/craftsmen), many of whom migrated from East Africa. Below these two major groups are the so-called 'outcaste' groups such as Bhatras (peddlars) and Chamars (leather workers) (Bhachu, 1985). To an outsider, it is very difficult to distinguish between these different groups. However, different caste groups can be recognised by family or clan name. Another pointer is the different styles of turban worn by men in different caste groups, as well as subtle differences in styles of dress. Among Sikhs in the UK, different caste groups will mix freely, work, eat and worship together. However, marriage between members of different castes is still taboo, although there are early signs that this situation may be changing as class (education, profession, wealth) rather than caste becomes more important among young Sikh professionals. Despite the fact that class has always existed within caste groups, the UK's social environment is making the idea of belonging to a specific caste group increasingly redundant.

Sikhism does not prescribe any days as being specifically auspicious or holy. Each day is seen as another opportunity to praise the creator and develop a relationship with Him. However, Sikhs are particularly drawn together on their major festivals. These include the birthdays of the Gurus (Gurpurbs) and Baisakhi (creation of the Khalsa). These festivals are seen as an opportunity to reflect on the Gurus' teachings, Sikh history and sacrifice. Many Sikhs will wait to be baptised on Baisakhi day.

New challenges

The rapid advances in medicine and biology present new challenges for the Sikh faith. There is general agreement on topics such as euthanasia and the making of a living will. Life is seen as a gift from God, and an opportunity to strive for enlightenment. Illness, suffering and pain are a result of one's actions, in this or a previous life, and should be endured with moral courage and fortitude. The ultimate point of release from this life is the will of God (Hukam) and it should not be interfered with. The intentional death of an individual by, for example, lethal injection is forbidden.

However, on the subject of artificial prolonging of life, the argument is not so unequivocal. Some Sikhs may argue that in cases where further treatment to cure is seen as uncompassionate or medically ineffective, the artificial prolonging of life should not be encouraged and the patient be allowed to die naturally. In all instances, the duty of family, friends and medical practitioners is to do everything to alleviate suffering and also to provide emotional and spiritual support during the last stages of life.

Other issues such as genetic engineering and stem-cell research trigger lively debate among Sikhs and as yet no clear consensus has emerged on these issues. Most Sikhs will therefore continue to make personal choices on these matters.

Conclusions

Sikhism has come a long way in a short space of time. From the message that Guru Nanak preached over 500 years ago, it has now grown into a cohesive and powerful religion that still retains diversity within it. For most Sikhs, their religion is a journey in search of Truth and represents an opportunity to connect with the Creator and achieve liberation. It also signifies a life of high moral conduct, active service and righteous living.

Key points of *Chapter 7*

- Sikhism was founded by Guru Nanak about 500 years ago.
- It is an ardently monotheistic religion (single god) believing that God is beyond human comprehension and formless. Sikhs also believe in the divinity of the soul, cycle of birth and rebirth, karma and liberation of the soul through good deeds and meditation.
- The Guru Granth Sahib, the holy book, is the Sikh's perpetual guide and the epitome of the spiritual teachings of Sikhism. It is centre of focus at all Sikh ceremonies. The gurdwara is the central place of worship for Sikhs.
- Sikhism does not prescribe that any special rituals be performed when looking after sick patients close to death or at the point of death. Meditation and recitation of Sikh prayers are the only key requirements. Sick patients may wish recordings of Sikh scriptures to be played at their bedside.
- Advances in biology and medicine such as stem-cell research and genetic engineering present new challenges to Sikhs in terms of interpreting scriptures and teachings to form a consensus on these issues.

References

Bhachu P (1985) *Twice Migrants: East African Sikh Settlers in Britain.* Tavistock Publications, London

Buck PS (1987) From the Foreword to the *Translation of the Guru Granth Sahib* by Gopal Singh, p. XIX, Vol 1, 7th edn. Allied Publishers, New Delhi

Cole WO, Sambhi PS (1978) *The Sikhs: their Religious Beliefs and Practices.* Routledge & Keegan Paul, London

Field D (1914) *The Religion of the Sikhs*. John Murray, London

Gatrad AR, Jhutti-Johal J, Gill P, Sheikh A (2005) Sikh birth customs. *Arch Dis Child* **90**: 560–3

Singh D (1994) *Sikhism: a Comparative Study of its Theology and Mysticism*. 2nd edn. Singh Brothers, Amritsar

Singh K (1977) *A History of the Sikhs*. Vol 1. Oxford University Press, New Delhi, India

Singh P (1999) *The Sikhs*. John Murray Publishers, London

www.sikhs.org.uk (accessed 2005)

CHAPTER 8

Palliative care for Sikhs

*Rashid Gatrad, Hardev Notta, Sukhmeet Singh Panesar,
Erica Brown, Aziz Sheikh*

*The nature of God is a circle, of which the circle is everywhere and the
circumference is nowhere.*
Anon

To understand fully the needs of patients, it is important to have a basic
appreciation of their beliefs and the possible ways in which these outlooks may
affect health and health-seeking behaviour. A study by Addington-Hall (2003)
suggested that the inclusion of 'care of the dying' in the medical curriculum has
had some impact on improving terminal-care provision. We believe that this
concept could also be adopted for those from diverse cultures, such as those
from the Sikh faith, both in the UK and the rest of the world.

Our hope is that the information presented here will help facilitate a more
informed discussion with patients, their families and carers about how best
to meet individual patient needs. This understanding is important because,
although the largest Sikh communities are to be found in northern India, smaller
communities now exist in most parts of the world, including North America and
Europe. For example, the 2001 UK census showed that over 300,000 Sikhs now
live in England and Wales, with particularly high concentrations in the Southall
district of London and the Midlands (Office for National Statistics, 2001).

This chapter builds on the previous one (*Chapter 7*) by providing an
overview of practical issues that may be of relevance for the palliative care of
Sikh patients. It is important, however, to avoid stereotyping and to be aware
that each individual may follow their religion to a greater or lesser extent.

Rashid Gatrad, Hardev Notta, Sukhmeet Singh Panesar, Erica Brown, Aziz Sheikh

Symbols of Sikhism

The principal symbol of Sikhism is made up of two swords, symbolising the need to fight, if necessary, for what is right. Between these is a circle, a symbol that God is one and without beginning or end. At the centre is a two-edged sword called a Khanda, which gives its name to the symbol (*Figure 8.1*).

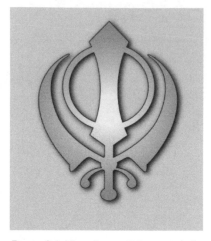

Figure 8.1 *Khanda, a religious symbol of Sikhism.*

The wearing of a turban is the most widely recognised symbol of Sikhism and helps to identify male members of the community. However, the assumption that someone is not a Sikh simply because he does not wear a turban should be avoided as some Sikhs have now abandoned this rite. Five symbols, also known as the 'Five Ks of Sikhism', characterise Sikhs (*Panel 8.1*). These symbols need to be respected. This is particularly important at the end of life, when, as with other faiths, attachment to religious symbols may assume heightened importance (Singh, 1977) (see *Introductory comment*, Section Two, by Gatrad and Gatrad).

Panel 8.1: The five Ks of Sikhism

- **Kara** — a bangle worn on the right wrist, which serves as a constant reminder of the faith.
- **Kesh** — uncut hair and hence the need for turbans for males.
- **Kanga** — a small wooden or plastic comb, denoting the importance of leading an ordered and disciplined life.
- **Kirpan** — a symbolic sword worn under the clothes, symbolising protection of the weak. In the UK, some Sikhs have a sword engraved on the side of a comb.
- **Katchera** — special underwear worn by both men and women, symbolising modesty and sexual morality. The leggings of such underwear may extend to the knees.

Care of the dying Sikh patient

Family ties

Providing for the emotional and spiritual well-being of relatives is believed by Sikhs to be a way of achieving unity with God. Although sons traditionally hold responsibility for the care and support of their ageing parents, more and more families need hospital/hospice care for their dying relatives. This reflects, in part, the continuing erosion of the extended family network.

Those requiring inpatient care can expect many visitors. Friends and relatives may recite Sikh hymns from the Guru Granth Sahib (the holy Sikh book) to console themselves and give comfort to the dying. A picture of a Guru may also be placed in the room as a reminder of Sikh teachings.

Hygiene and diet

Like Muslims and Hindus, a shower is preferred to a bath, as stagnant water is considered unhygienic, particularly before prayers. The availability of a water jug in toilets is often greatly appreciated. Some Sikhs are vegetarian; halaal and kosher meats are forbidden and most Sikhs will not eat beef. Observant Sikhs may be offended if offered alcohol or alcohol-containing foods.

Role of prayers

Devout Sikhs often rise early to pray. Supplications continue throughout the day, with Mala (a string of prayer beads) often used as an adjunct, just as Catholics may use rosary beads. Patients sometimes use holy water called Amrit. This is made up in the Gurdwara (the Sikh place of worship), consists of sugar and water, and is drunk. Occasionally, this water is brought from Amritsar in India. Amrit is a sacred institution of the Sikh way of life, denoting a willingness to live and die for God and it is therefore important that this water is treated with respect; in particular, staff should be made aware that it is not to be inadvertently discarded. The Gutka (book of prayers) should not be touched with unwashed hands. It is best stored on a high shelf.

Rashid Gatrad, Hardev Notta, Sukhmeet Singh Panesar, Erica Brown, Aziz Sheikh

The time of death

As a result of the belief in the doctrine of Karma (reincarnation, depending on one's past deeds), some Sikhs, in particular the elderly, will accept death stoically. At death, those present are encouraged to exclaim 'Waheguru!' ('Wonderful Lord!'). Eyes are closed and the limbs straightened. The family will wash and dress the body. Yoghurt is sometimes used in the washing, as it is considered a good cleansing agent. The deceased is typically dressed in a white cotton shroud (although red may be used for younger women) with the five Ks, and taken home so that family and friends have the opportunity to pay their final respects (Seth, 1970).

Issues after death

Children and adults are cremated, whereas those stillborn or dying in early infancy are buried. The male relative has the honour of igniting the fire during cremations, although in Western countries this role is replaced symbolically by pressing the button of the curtains surrounding the coffin in the crematorium. Both males and females attend cremations. The ashes may be scattered into local rivers, but some families will return to the Punjab and scatter them in the River Sutlej in Anandpur, which marks the birthplace of Sikhism.

Post-mortems and transplant requests

Post-mortem examinations are generally discouraged. This relates to the belief that the dead person has suffered enough. The family do not generally cook food until after cremation, which, if delayed, could mean providing accommodation for many relatives and friends.

As the Sikh religion encourages helping others in need, donating one's organs is considered a noble gesture and transplant teams need not have any particular anxieties about approaching Sikh patients or their families to discuss this matter.

Bereavement

Although there is no specific period of mourning, it is usual for it to last ten to fifteen days. Crying is discouraged during this period and at other times, and the bereaved are encouraged to accept the will of God (see *Chapter 15* for a more detailed discussion of bereavement).

Conclusions

We have in this chapter aimed to provide some practical advice on improving understanding and communication with Sikh patients and their families as they seek terminal care. We have attempted to emphasise that palliation should include not only the care of a patient's body, but also his or her soul. In the case of Sikhs, this may involve appreciation of the sense and significance of their karma or destiny. To this end the understanding of giving both physical and spiritual 'space' to the patient and his or her relatives is crucial. They should be allowed to carry on their cultural rituals in a sympathetic environment, without being embarrassed or criticised. It is only when this happens with cultures that are different from those in the West that diversity will have its true meaning, take root and grow in strength.

Key points of *Chapter 8*

- The main religious book for Sikhs is the Guru Granth Sahib.
- Sikhs believe in karma (ie. reincarnation), depending on one's deeds.
- The most important symbols of Sikhism are the five Ks.
- Clinicians should try to ensure that there is no gender error as male Sikhs without turbans often have long hair.
- Holy water is called Amrit and should be treated with respect.
- Halaal and kosher foods should not be offered to Sikhs.
- Both children and adults are cremated, although babies may be buried.

References

Addington-Hall J (2003) Care of the dying: end of life care needs start-of-career training. *Hospital Doctor* **13 March**: 20–5

Chan KP, Pickering M, Pai S, Sheikh A, Soloman A (2003) Doctors and their faith. *BMJ* **326**: S135–8

Channa BS, Murbah JS (1984) *The Sikh Gurus and Brief Glimpses of the Sikh Way of Life*. East African Ramgarhia Board, Nairobi

Gatrad AR, Sheikh A (2002a) Palliative care for Muslims and issues before death. *Int J Palliat Nurs* **8**: 526–31

Gatrad AR, Sheikh A (2002b) Palliative care for Muslims and issues after death. *Int J Palliat Nurs* **8**: 594–7

Gatrad AR, Choudhary P, Sheikh A (2003) Palliative care for Hindus. *Int J Palliat Nurs* **9**: 442–8

Office for National Statistics (ONS) (2001) www.statistics.gov.uk/census2001 (accessed 2005)

Seth VP (1970) *Guru Nanak: Nanak is with the Lowliest*. Asia Press, Delhi

Sidhu GS (1973) *A Brief Introduction to Sikhism*. Sikh Missionary Society, Middlesex

Singh T (1977) *The Turban and the Sword of the Sikhs*. Sikh Missionary Society, Middlesex

Section Three:
Delivering Care

Improving communication and access to palliative care through the arts

Dipti P Thakker, Christina Faull

Ethnic minority populations frequently have less access to information and commonly experience a sense of disempowerment in their interaction with statutory services. Specific strategies are needed for this.

Commission for Racial Equality, UK

Severe illnesses such as cancer are often regarded as taboo subjects for discussion within South-Asian cultures, sometimes even within the family unit. Thus, discussions with health professionals about death and dying, especially from cancer, may be fraught with difficulties. Health education and health promotion therefore require not only careful consideration of cultural issues, but standard methodology, which requires appropriate adaptation. The most vulnerable groups are harder to target with lifestyle interventions, as they speak very little English and are relatively isolated from mainstream society with variable knowledge and motivation to use conventional health services.

In most parts of the Indian subcontinent, there is no concept of palliative care and if one considers that palliative care is basically a Western concept with no direct translation into any South-Asian language, it is hardly surprising that there is poor knowledge amongst South Asians of such services.

A lack of knowledge and information about palliative-care services contributes to the low uptake of cancer and palliative services amongst South Asian and other minority ethnic groups (Hill and Penso, 1995). Although there appear to be more similarities than differences in the needs people have for support and symptom management, members of ethnic-minority communities still do not adequately access services to meet these needs (Faull, 2003). This is partly because such services do not exist, but more commonly because patients and their families are not aware of them, or they are thought to be inappropriate by some GPs, who feel that people from South-Asian communities have little grasp of the concept of palliative care. Therefore, patients and families often fail to benefit from such services.

It has been suggested that traditional methods of health education and health promotion in the UK that include presentations, lectures and leaflets are culturally inappropriate for many South-Asian communities (Thakker, 2000). Such methods are often ineffective because of language barriers or, even with successful communication, they lead to information being regarded as irrelevant due to the didactic nature of message delivery. Raising awareness of sensitive health issues such as cancer and palliative care requires delivery that needs to be adapted to overcome cultural taboos and long-held beliefs.

In this chapter, we describe an initiative using the arts in the West Midlands, UK, that aimed to engage South Asians in discussions about cancer and dying, with concomitant information on palliative-care services in the hope that such innovation could foster links between palliative-care services and local communities. It was a cyclical process of collecting data, reflecting on it and feeding it back explicitly and proactively to participants, who included clinicians, managers, community workers and service users. This reflective methodology was educational for both us and the participants.

Communicating through the arts

Art speaks to us and addresses our emotional and spiritual needs. Art of any kind arises in the artist's mind and therefore will be affected by his or her beliefs and values. Patients with cancer and other terminal illness have often used the written and visual arts to convey their experiences. These have had a huge influence on others with cancer, on health policy and on individual health practitioners. Examples include:

- *The Emotional Cancer Journey* (2003) by Michele Petrone (art and poetry)
- *The Diving Bell and the Butterfly* (1997) by Jean-Dominique Bauby (a memoir)
- *Whose Life is it Anyway?* (1978) by Brian Clark (a play)
- *A Very Easy Death* (1969) by Simone de Beauvoir (a memoir).

Arts and health have a creative tension in their relationship. Health care is perceived as predominantly based on scientific evidence, largely addressing the physical needs of people. Arts, on the other hand, are perhaps at their best when challenging old ideas and taking novel direction. They target primarily the emotional, spiritual and sensory dimensions of being alive. Such different emphases have an important and growing role in health. They have certainly been shown to be effective in health promotion, influencing health behaviours and health strategy in mental-health services when used as an integral part of healthcare delivery (Halldane and Loppert, 1999).

South Asian Palliative Care Awareness Arts (SAPCAA) project

Arts such as film, dance, music, drawing, storytelling and poetry have a significant place in all South-Asian cultures and the South Asian Palliative Care Awareness Arts (SAPCAA) project grew from recognition of the importance of this influence within these communities. The project incorporated artists and doctors whose aim was to improve the care of South Asian cancer patients and their families in the West Midlands by providing culturally relevant information about coping with advanced cancer and helping patients improve their lives during terminal care. The project was based at the University Hospital NHS Trust in Birmingham and funded by the New Opportunities Fund as a part of the 'Living with Cancer' initiative.

SAPCAA recognised the potential of the arts not only in helping engage patients and families from a diverse range of backgrounds, but also in helping them overcome barriers of language and taboos associated with people suffering from cancer in South-Asian communities. Preliminary work identified a comfortable forum allowing people to relate their own stories of personal and sensitive experiences through creative and performance arts. Both live drama and the use of film were found to stimulate audience participation in discussions and encourage a sharing of experiences, particularly of unmet needs.

A wide spectrum of art forms were used and participation was encouraged, irrespective of gender or age, from members of diverse South-Asian communities across the West Midlands. The principles were:

- you learn best from being able to relate directly to the way the subject is presented
- you learn best when enjoying
- you learn best from people you can relate to
- you learn best from participating.

Specifically commissioning a drama that could reach out to the communities, the SAPCAA project manager worked with the artists and took advice from community organisations and professionals involved in palliative care and facilitated the many events and classes to improve understanding of palliative care. The artists and community workers themselves eventually became the main educators about palliative care to their own communities.

SAPCAA set up three different community arts projects: each worked at a grass-roots level and involved different South-Asian religious groups based on the preferences of the identified groups of artists, health professionals and community members.

For each project the artists themselves undertook workshop training in palliative care and were able to discuss palliative care with participants at their own pace and so develop a sensitive appreciation of the cultural taboos associated with discussing cancer, death and dying. Furthermore, the artists were to help participants create artwork that reflected awareness of palliative care.

Each project provided a forum for discussion and an opportunity to collate attitudes to cancer and palliative care using focus-group methodology. These classes also provided an opportunity for participants to use their newly acquired skills to pass on knowledge of palliative care to their own community. The three projects (discussed below) were:

- creative arts
- disk jockey
- school drama workshop

The creative arts project

A textile artist offered teaching to participants on painting and embroidery skills. The participants were all female and mainly elderly. They learnt about palliative care and transmitted this in their beautiful work (*Figures 9.1–9.3*). The paintings were placed in hospices through an auction in which the paintings were sponsored by a South-Asian businessman. They discussed issues of fear and ignorance associated with hospices and stressed the needs of cancer patients and their carers:

'I am so proud of my paintings; my experience of my brother dying in front of my eyes is still there. There are no places like what the ladies have talked about back home.'

'These classes have helped me to learn of a care we could all get — my work will take pride in a hospice.'

'These pictures placed in hospices will make our people feel at home.'

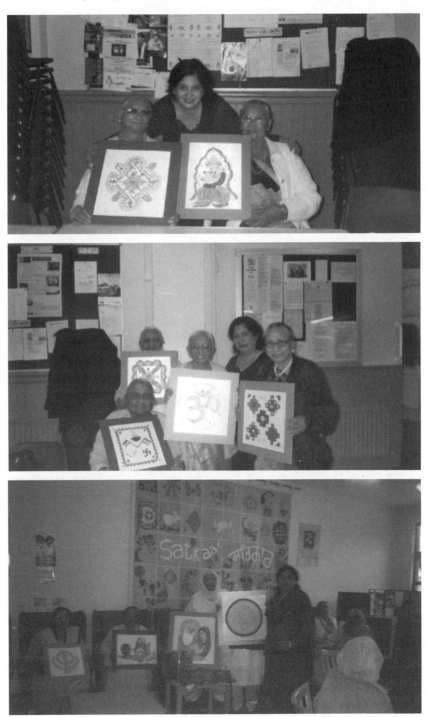

Figures 9.1–9.3: Patients display the work they produced with the help of a textile artist on a creative arts project.

The Disk Jockey (DJ) project

Cultural norms dictate that many young South Asians become carers. It is important that they are aware of the support they can receive. However, as it is difficult to engage young people in learning key health messages through traditional educational settings, SAPCAA created a novel approach for this group. The DJ project was based within a community centre that was already popular for providing extra-curricular learning opportunities for South-Asian youth. After undertaking the SAPCAA palliative care workshop, a DJ facilitated teaching and discussion of cancer and palliative care within a 'DJ skills' course. In addition, these DJ students learnt about palliative care through a specially developed short drama that focused on the experiences of young carers of terminally ill patients. The students were asked to organise an end of course drama to pass on their knowledge of palliative care through their DJ'ing skills. Families and friends came to see them perform 'raps' (short musical lyrics) through which they conveyed their thoughts on palliative care (see end of chapter).

Schools drama workshop project

The drama sketch used in the DJ project was found to be a powerful way of relaying information on palliative care and in engaging participants in discussion. This drama was used in a series of workshops at secondary schools across the West Midlands. The actors who contributed to the drama workshop found the work important and educational. They remarked:

> *'Palliative care is great to work on. I have learnt many aspects of palliative care — for example, the emotions a family can go through and how this can be helped by the Macmillan nurses.'*

> *'I have been doing [researching] palliative care for about a week. Performing it as an actor has made me realise what impact it has on families. It's been an interesting topic to work on.'*

Palliative care awareness events

SAPCAA produced its own thirty-minute video drama called *Humara Safar* (Our Journey) in Hindi with English subtitles. This drama portrays the experiences of a

South-Asian family with an elderly member suffering with advanced cancer. The story identifies the difficulties faced by the family and positively highlights both the types of services and the benefits the family received from using palliative-care services. Day-care and home-care teams from the hospice and district and Marie Curie and Macmillan nurses are all portrayed in these videos.

These healthcare events were supported by local palliative-care services. Such events have gained popularity amongst health promotion specialists due to their ability, through health stalls, to promote and simultaneously educate a relatively large number of people. We used music, dance, drama, food and associated activities such as fashion shows at events hosted in popular community venues to raise awareness about palliative care. For some events, transport was provided. This encouraged large-scale participation by targeted communities. The events centred on the showing of the *Humara Safar* video drama and were well-attended; in Coventry, for example, a crowd in excess of 500 people attended; a hospice in Wolverhampton had eighty people visit from local South-Asian communities.

One of the objectives of SAPCAA was to increase the understanding by health providers and commissioners of the needs of South-Asian communities. This was not easy because of lack of motivation, perceived irrelevance for such type of discussion, and cultural appropriateness of this type of approach. Discussions were however facilitated by the video drama, which not only motivated people to talk and voice their opinion, but also encouraged in-depth discussions and expressions of unmet needs by participants with personal experiences of those suffering from cancer:

'The doctor never does anything. They think we are always coming to them with small problem.'

'I know a lady who went to her doctor so many times of something wrong with her breast, but he said there was nothing wrong. She died of cancer...'

'GPs should help us more. If they do not tell us, it is sometimes difficult for us to ask — most of them do not have time or still do nothing even if you ask!'

The identified needs varied according to the individual and their profession or roles. For example, link workers identified 'talking to someone' as a key need with 'more health workers required from the South-Asian culture'. On the other hand, lay persons identified the following needs:

- care in the home
- more benefits
- more information (verbal and written)
- information from the GP
- lack of bereavement support (frequently highlighted in the workshops)
- advice and direction.

Evaluation of the SAPCAA project

Evaluation, through questionnaires distributed to a randomly selected sample of attendees, conducted at the events were very positive. The samples of quotations below highlight the success in informing participants of all ages and from different communities about the relevance of palliative care. The powerful storyline of the drama encouraged discussion and a sharing of experiences:

'*The drama brought tears my eyes. My family had told our father of his cancer in the garden, just as shown in the story.*'

'*It is the care we can all get for us or someone of ours who is suffering from an illness with no cure.*'

'*You know for the first time we are seeing people talking, asking questions and sharing their personal stories – it is normally not easy to do this.*'

'*… the video was very sentimental; it taught me so much about cancer.*'

'*Events like this should happen more often, we enjoy and learn so much!*'

A young boy asked for a copy of the video. When asked why he should want a copy, as he was quite young to make the request, he replied:

'*My mother is not here at the event because she has cancer and did not want to come. But I wanted her to see the video, please — is that okay?*'

We believe that this video has been a powerful tool in raising awareness about palliative care, as it began to motivate people to help change their local services. Many carers and patients amongst the participants sought further guidance. One example is an elderly Hindu lady who was very concerned because she was recently told that her daughter could have cancer. Having spoken to the Cancer Link Nurse of her family's needs, she said, 'At least I know what to ask for and who to ask.'

Through questionnaire-based evaluation and verbal feedback from focus groups, the project was able to collate data on perceptions of attitudes to palliative care and services. These data showed that the concept of palliative care is not widely recognised in South-Asian communities. We confirmed that the word 'palliative' was an unfamiliar term for many lay South-Asian people and, surprisingly, this was also the case amongst some non-medical and non-nursing health professionals. However, many palliative-care providers have also raised such concerns for other communities who may or may not be more familiar with the concepts and ethos of palliative care than South-Asian communities appear to be.

We found that most South-Asian people had not heard of hospices and if they had, they were thought to be either 'a Christian rest home' or 'an old people's home'. One person commented:

'Tell me why there is still a Christian feel to the hospices? Our people are not going to feel comfortable there. You do not even have any Asian staff.'

This finding indicates a potential barrier to uptake of hospice services. Other barriers identified in discussions were:

- the hospice was seen as a place to die
- not a custom in South-Asian culture
- not suited to individual needs.

Many members of South-Asian cultures take pride and regard it their duty to 'look after their own', in particular the elderly. If hospices are thought of as rest homes, and services are not seen as supporting their particular needs, then services may not be favoured. Aspects of day-care services and 'hospice at home service' would be important benefits to highlight when promoting palliative services.

Once understood, palliative-care services were perceived to be important. Information provided was seen to be of use 'to inform others in need,' 'to help people with cancer' and 'to know where to get help'. Many people perceived information to be personally relevant and identified the support of the service as being beneficial.

The majority of the students in both the DJ and schools drama workshops projects had not heard of palliative care. The projects appeared to give students a clearer understanding of the philosophy of palliative-care services:

'It takes some stress off the family.'

'It helps the person with cancer and his family go through and cope with all sorts of problems, including emotional stress.'

'It provides "space" in which the family of the terminally ill person can get some rest and time away from emotional stress.'

Conclusions

All three projects clearly showed how the arts could be used to deliver knowledge of a sensitive subject to all age-groups through focused activities that engage participants. The key to success appeared to be methods that were fun and stimulating, thereby facilitating learning.

In the creative arts project, we found that within the comfortable environment of the classes the discussions that took place highlighted a wish by the participants to express unmet needs through sharing past experiences. This project also showed how participants, once motivated by knowledge, wished to help contribute to and change services. The donation of the paintings to hospices by participants can be taken as an example of an indirect and culturally appropriate way of the participants getting involved with improving services. Sponsorship of paintings by local South-Asian businessmen is also an example of a culturally appropriate way of South-Asian communities getting involved with palliative-care service provision. Furthermore, the creative arts project provided a platform for hospices to continue user involvement and obtain support from local South-Asian communities. Through continued liaison with sponsors and artists, the hospices can obtain advice on how to tackle sensitive cultural issues, eradicate stigmas associated with hospice care, and improve recruitment of staff from South-Asian communities.

Our experiences indicate the success of the use of art in palliative care — in particular, the use of drama to deliver knowledge of not only a sensitive subject, but also one that consists of words such as 'palliative' for which there is no direct translation in any South-Asian language. Children from South-Asian communities often have a role in bringing home important health-related information to other family members. Empowering them may help improve awareness of palliative care, not only for the family but also for the community.

The arts engaged and united people from a diverse range of cultural, ethnic and religious backgrounds and professions. The drama and the events reached out to people from other groups such as the African Caribbean and the Yemeni community. For some health professionals, the format of the events, as well as the media used, have been educational with respect to furthering understanding of cultural diversity; an unintended, but nonetheless welcome, consequence of this has been that our video is now used for diversity training sessions.

Music and dance were used to encourage people to attend events and were appreciated by all South-Asian communities. The incorporation of health education was a success, since the project brought a new dimension to the use of arts in this way. Many of the artists not only learned about palliative care themselves, but were also motivated in continuing to use the arts for other aspects of health education. As South-Asian artists are presently few and far between, they are usually well-known amongst the local communities and therefore could prove to be an excellent vehicle for transfer of information. The project has also introduced creative activities offered by the artists to the day-care units at hospices and oncology wards.

In summary, the SAPCAA project highlighted the effectiveness of working at a grass-roots level to encourage participation of communities in health education that helps tackle cultural barriers that otherwise lead to inequalities in health.

B-Gyalz rap lyrics

Now here's a story all about how
My life got quipped all upside down
And I'd like to take a minute
Just sitting right there and tell you how
I became a client of palliative care

I found out I was soon to die
Shocked, shaken, not a cry
A little old lady knocked on the door
Palliative care, tell me more
She started off blabbing on about the crap
Thought she looked so ugly, she needed a slap

Then I realised how important it was
The help was available totally class
Nursing, considerations, take your pick
Awareness attentions all at a click
Getting real bad
Showing it aint sad
The emptiness or the pain

Without care for life's unbearable, the prospects
Unthinkable

Trouble started off, my family
Found out
Daughters kicked doors
Son began to shout
Wife was there looking all bleak
I felt the anxiety, concerned and weak

Little old lady came back the next day
Was caring, comforting and told me to pray
I was so scared I asked her to stay
She sat there, said she'd do as I say

I told her, 'Go talk to my son'
She jumped right up all for one
All gentle and moderate, as bright as the sun
As good as gold like a nun
They both went out to another room
I was still shaking, my heart went boom

I felt so daint, feel like I wasa dying
Da pain was gone I felt like crying
Then realised da gals and da wife
Waitin' der all in strife

Da gals went runnin', 'We don't want him to die'
Da wife opened up and gave out a loud cry
The l'il old lady just looked up tender
She was so comforting, no matter what the gender
Her being there
Showing that she cares
I was so glad, didn't care about the fears
The contention, dissention, friction had all gone
Her thoughtfulness, cautiousness, people's choice of fun
I thought even though she probably didn't care
I looked at her face
She looked with a glare
It was as if she was telling me,
'Yes, I do care'

I realised there wasn't much left to do
I was dying, it was more scary than true
L'il old lady still there to use
I called her up and told her the news
She was so gentle
'It's not the end yet'
'Yes it is, I'm ready and set'
While I was saying that I felt my heart content
A voice inside me saying, 'There's quality time to be spent'

Key points of *Chapter 9*

- In South-Asian communities, death and dying do not necessarily have to be taboo subjects.
- Given an appropriate stimulus and a comfortable forum, the subject of death can be readily discussed and personal experiences shared.
- Health events interspersed with arts are a good mode of health education for both younger and older generations in South-Asian communities.
- A drama with a powerful storyline can enable people to relate to health experiences such as living with cancer, grasping new health concepts and perceiving the relevance of health services.
- A project aiming to raise awareness of any health subject needs to reach out by working at grass-roots level and motivating individual members of communities to become proactive in health promotion to their own communities.
- Such information can inform local and national policy of the plight of South Asians who require palliative care.

References

Bauby JD (1997) *The Diving Bell and the Butterfly*. Fourth Estate, London

Clarke B (1978) *Whose Life is it Anyway?* Amber Lane Press, Ashover, Derbyshire

De Beauvoir SO (1969) *A Very Easy Death*. Transl. Penguin, London

Faull C (2003) Cancer and palliative care. In: Kai J (ed) *Ethnicity, Health and Primary Care*. Oxford University Press, Oxford

Halldane D, Loppert A (1999) *The Arts in Health Care: Learning from Experience*. King's Fund, London

Hill D, Penso D (1995) *Opening Doors: Improving Access to Hospices and Specialist Palliative Care Services by the Members of the Black and Ethnic Minority Communities*. National Council for Hospice and Specialist Palliative Care Services, London

Petrone MA (2003) *The Emotional Cancer Journey*. MAP Foundation, London (www.mapfoundation.org)

Thakker D (2000) Attitudes to and Perceptions of Cancer in South Asian Women. MSc thesis. University of Southampton, Southampton

CHAPTER 10

South-Asian mothers with a life-limited child at Acorns Children's Hospices

Erica Brown

I expect to pass through this world but once, therefore any good that I can do or any kindness that I can show to any fellow creature, let me do it now; let me not defer it or neglect it, for I shall not pass this way again.
Stephen Grellett (1773–1855)

As a parent, it is a shattering experience to accept what is unacceptable — the news that your child has a life-limiting illness. Several authors write about the isolation that parents face as they struggle to come to terms with their shock (Hornby, 1994; Carpenter, 1997). There may be several phases in a child's illness, extending from the time of diagnosis through various treatments and relapses until there is an indication that curative therapy is not a viable option. For most families, loss begins at the time their child's life-limiting condition is disclosed — this is no different for South-Asian families. The task of coping for these parents is a process in which they find themselves constantly adjusting to the new demands that their ill child makes.

During the last decade, parental bereavement has received considerable attention and a number of studies have brought to light the unique needs of life-limited children and their families (Brown, 2002; Goldman, 2002; Hill, 1994). However, while there is an abundance of literature available on the psychological needs of families with a life-limited child, scant attention has been paid to cultural issues (Irish, Lundquist and Nelson, 1999), in particular the experiences and expectations of South-Asian families with a life-limited child.

There is sometimes a stereotype-driven simplification or assumption that the needs of families from ethnic-minority groups are met by resources from within their own community (Atkins and Rollings, 1998). However, evidence shows that, as they usually do not come forward for help, their needs are often unmet and they struggle with little support (Firth, 2001; NHS Executive, 2000). Therefore, the need to provide accessible and appropriate palliative care to ethnic-minority groups has been recognised as a significant service-development priority. A report from the National Council for Hospice and Specialist Palliative Care Services (Hill and Penso, 1995) identified, among other issues, a need for the provision of culturally sensitive services in relation to the 'spiritual, language and dietary needs of black and ethnic-minority service users'.

In the UK, about 15,000 children require palliative care each year. Many of them will receive care from a children's hospice, either in the community or in a hospice building. There are currently thirty-four children's hospices in the UK with several others in the planning stages. At Acorns in Birmingham, over 30% of usage is by children and families from South-Asian backgrounds. Children's hospices offer flexible, family-centred support throughout the course of a child's illness, and after death.

Overall mortality for the 14.8 million children and young adults aged zero to nineteen years with a life-limiting condition is as high as 1.9 per 10,000. It is therefore estimated that roughly three thousand children die each year from a life-limiting condition (Association for Children with Life-threatening or Terminal Conditions [ACT], 2003).

Since South Asians have proportionately greater numbers of young people compared with white communities, the number of children requiring palliative care from these communities is rising and will continue to do so for the foreseeable future (Hatton *et al*, 2004).

A unique feature of palliative care for children is the wide spectrum of conditions that may render a child in need of such care. ACT and the Royal College of Paediatrics and Child Health (1997) identified four broad groups of children likely to require palliative care (see *Chapter 11, Panel 11.1*). Most of the South-Asian children that Acorns Children's Hospices care for are from the last three categories, suggesting that, for the moment at least, cancer is not the commonest reason for palliative care.

A number of UK government publications (Department of Health [DoH], 1997, 1998; Scottish Office, 1997; Welsh Office, 1998) recommend that the views of patients and families are included in planning care that children with life-limiting illnesses receive. Historically, families with a disabled child have been excluded from policies aimed at improving quality of life (Connors and Stalker, 2003). However, families of a life-limited child have a range of needs that change as the illness progresses. For families from ethnic-minority groups, their needs are much more diverse and, nationally, largely unmet.

Although families and professionals may have differing perceptions of disease, their expertise and insights are complementary. Such interaction is crucial if the quality of palliative care is to be optimised. At the onset of a child's illness, parents will not have the same knowledge about a life-limiting condition as the professionals. However, as they assimilate more and more information, their understanding and grasp of both the physical and psychological impact of disease and its treatment on their child often surpasses that of clinicians. Therefore, parents are best-placed to know their child's likes and dislikes, in addition to how best to communicate with them and comfort them in culturally specific ways. They also have considerable insight into their own aims and values; their skills and knowledge; their strengths, weaknesses and difficulties. Indeed, they are the only people who can decide what they want for their child and family. Family-based palliative care is therefore an effective and preferred option for many families.

Because hospice care is a philosophy, not a facility, support can be provided in a number of settings. This chapter focuses on the experiences of South-Asian mothers who have a child with a life-limiting condition and their hopes and expectations for the care they will receive during their child's life.

Caring for South Asian children and families — the Acorns Children's Hospice model (Birmingham, UK)

The fundamental element of quality healthcare services are that provision is accessible to all users — it should be relevant to the health needs of the local population and provided in a manner socially and culturally acceptable to users in the community. At Acorns, we believe that we are able to meet client needs through making a valuable contribution to holistic family care. Work within the organisation has always sought to engage families fully so that policy and practice complement each other.

For professionals to address the needs of ethnic minorities, they should not only be aware of the need to be culturally sensitive, but also understand that practices, beliefs and attitudes are constantly changing with acculturation; thus, the cultural values of the host population are having an increasing influence on those of minority groups.

Acorns Children's Hospices provide a network of community-based and hospice-based care for life-limited children and their families throughout the West Midlands, Shropshire, Staffordshire, Warwickshire, Herefordshire, Worcestershire and Gloucestershire. Among these families, there are a large number of clients from South-Asian cultures. The service model includes employing community workers, a sibling worker, care staff and volunteers from different ethnic communities. At a time when many other children's hospices are finding it difficult to attract referrals from minority ethnic groups, the number of families using Acorns who are members of South-Asian communities is increasing. This would appear to result from a commitment towards family care and opportunities for staff and volunteer training that are integral to the service provided, rather than additional to everyday practice. Central to our success have been the appointment of an Asian Liaison Officer; recruitment of volunteers through placing advertisements in appropriate languages; and the formation of an Asian Mother Support Group.

Disclosure of diagnosis

The importance of providing accurate and accessible information for families (particularly when English is not a first language) has been emphasised in a number of studies (for example, Mir *et al*, 2001). The manner in which diagnosis of their child's life-limiting illness was disclosed to the family has been shown to play a significant part in how well individual family members adapt (Brown, 2001). So often parents are confronted with a medical diagnosis that is unfamiliar to them, and professionals have seldom considered this. This means that parents may be left without professional support and with unanswered questions concerning their child's condition. With difficulties of communication and access, this scenario is worse for South Asians and other minority ethnic groups.

Meeting the challenge

In 2003, Acorns Children's Hospices carried out a small-scale research project that set out to understand the experiences and expectations of South-Asian mothers with a life-limited child using our services. A summary of findings is presented in *Panel 10.1* and *Panel 10.2* with a subsequent discussion of these issues in the hope that there are clear messages that could in turn inform future strategy of palliative services for South-Asian families.

Because mothers did not always have detailed information about their child's life expectancy and the implications of this for their family, many were unsure where to access ongoing support. Others described feeling suffocated by the constant flurry of clinic and hospital appointments, and the intensity of the emotions they felt.

Our research showed that once a diagnosis was made, all South-Asian mothers experienced anxiety relaying the information to extended-family members. Significantly, several mothers had struggled to break the news to their own parents. Although the impact of different communication styles within families has been widely researched (Tasker, 1998), open communication,

Panel 10.1: Experiences of South-Asian mothers after their child was diagnosed with a life-limiting condition

■ There was a long interval between the first and subsequent appointments.

■ Disclosure was by a paediatric consultant and in English.

■ Written information was given in less than half the cases.

■ Half the mothers believed that their child had a disability and not a life-limiting condition.

■ There was no consistency in the explanations because mothers subsequently saw different doctors.

■ None of the mothers felt that they had received sufficient professional support in the days and weeks following the disclosure.

■ Being able to talk to other Asian women with a life-limited child through the Acorns Asian Mothers Group was tremendously important for mothers. Sharing experiences and concerns in group-work situations helped to relieve the sense of isolation mothers felt within their families.

■ Some mothers recounted incidents when they had experienced negative responses from people in their local community. These occasions ranged from being avoided by mothers with well children; being denied access to a shop with a wheelchair; being stared at; and being spoken about as 'the mother with the mental child'.

■ Although interpreters were deemed useful, they did not have much insight into life-limiting illnesses.

■ Information about available services written in relevant languages was important to the families.

■ Families experienced enormous anxiety about the transition from paediatric palliative-care services to adult palliative care.

■ Mothers were unanimous in expressing a wish for help with household chores so that they could spend quality time with their life-limited child.

■ Several mothers suffered poor physical health themselves and would value help in lifting their child or carrying out personal-care tasks in their own home such as bathing, feeding, toileting and dressing.

■ Mothers reported that they suffered a high rate of health-related problems. Whilst most of the interviewees talked in depth about physical problems, such as tiredness, backache (from lifting their child), headache and stomach problems, they also referred to 'being exhausted', 'worried', 'depressed' and 'feeling constantly anxious'.

■ Most mothers who were interviewed said they were unable to leave their child unattended unless the child was asleep.

■ In addition to having a restricted social life themselves, mothers said that they felt that their life-limited child had limited opportunities to interact with well children. *[continues...]*

> **Panel 10.1 [continued]: Experiences of South-Asian mothers after their child was diagnosed with a life-limiting condition**
>
> - The majority of families had not been able to take a holiday during the last three years. They didn't feel able to leave their child in respite care at the hospice, as two weeks was not long enough for a visit to their country of origin.
> - Contrary to expectation, most mothers reported that there was no support from the extended family.
> - Although there were no marriage break-downs, there were great tensions between the different in-laws.

characterised by families being honest with each other, has been found to enhance the coping strategies of parents; those in control of their own emotions are generally able to communicate with other members of their family (Fanos and Weiner, 1994). In this context, a rare remark from a mother was:

> *'We don't have to hide things any more. If my daughter is ill, I tell our family why'.*

Often, families turned to their faith to find a reason for why their child was sick or to provide comfort in facing what lay ahead. Some mothers said that their faith was important to them, although some gave examples of being marginalised by their religious community, especially if the place of worship was not readily accessible or if their child made a noise.

Support services available to mothers included education, health, social services and the children's hospice. The significant negative factor in mothers' views was the poor collaboration between the service providers they used, an issue described in previous research studies (Quinton, 2004). Chamba *et al*'s (1999) study revealed that South-Asian families with a disabled child had high levels of awareness of general health and welfare services, but much lower awareness of support agencies providing respite care, counselling and psychological support. At Acorns, all the mothers were aware of what was available to them, but this was largely expected, since each family had a dedicated community worker from the hospice, part of whose role included helping parents access services or negotiate access on their behalf. Where mothers had used support services, some of these had been deemed by them to be culturally inappropriate, particularly in relation to language and gender issues, a finding supported by Hatton *et al*'s (2004) study of South-Asian families with a disabled child. One mother remarked:

**Panel 10.2: Education of South-Asian children
with life-limiting conditions**

- All of the mothers with children of school age were able to take advantage of education. Most children attended special schools.
- Overall parents were very pleased with the education services their child received, feeling that the curriculum offered was appropriate to their child's cognitive development.
- Generally, parents felt their child's cultural and religious needs were well met by schools, and were delighted to find that care assistants were often the same gender as their child. Schools provided parents with valuable opportunities for respite during term time.
- In all families, the child's statement of Special Educational Needs had been explained well by the Local Education Authority (LEA) and parents had been able to have an interpreter present to explain how the school would meet their child's needs.
- The majority of mothers interviewed with a school-age child felt that their child enjoyed education.

'The counsellor was Asian, and although she spoke the same language as I do, she talked in English all the time. I can't think in English when I'm telling her upsetting things'.

Although most of the mothers did not express a preference for support services to be staffed by South Asians, it was important to all mothers that, if they approached a service or paid a visit, their main contact person was female.

Respite care is an important feature of the supportive care that a family receives. The UK Parliamentary Select Committee Inquiry Report, *Recommendations into Palliative Care* (21 July, 2004), calls for an increase in palliative and respite care services for young adults. In independent evaluations of children's hospice care, parents have consistently valued the support provided (Bradshaw and Webb, 1997; Nash, 1998; Phillips and Burt, 1999). Other than respite provided by school, most parents were not able to enjoy a break, apart from staying at Acorns Children's Hospices.

'I haven't seen my mother since my wedding seventeen years ago. I can't go to see her even though she is getting old, because there is nobody to take care of my children. I feel I can leave my son at the hospice, but I need twenty-one days of care for him and they are only able to offer me fourteen. Other mothers need their child cared for here as well'.

Professionals and policy-makers have a key role in supporting the welfare and continuity of education for children with life-limiting illnesses. Research by Closs and Norris (1997) highlighted the fact that many life-limited children and those with chronic medical conditions were unable to access the kind of support that would benefit their education. Our parents were very positive about the education their child received (*Panel 10.2*).

'School helps to make life normal — such a good time for Gurpreet'.

The numbers of life-limited young people from South-Asian families cared for permanently outside their home are not known. Evidence from the 2001 UK Census suggests that young disabled adults from South-Asian families are more than 50% more likely to be cared for in residential settings compared with their white counterparts (Office National Statistics [ONS], 2001). Some parents felt let down by the service:

'They offered me a lifeline and then they took it away. It is hard because when he was at residential school, I had some respite — but now he is seventeen he is with me all the time. After school finishes, it seems like that really will be the end of everything. Then we just wait for the time for him to die'.

Generally, the coping strategies employed by mothers changed at different stages of their child's illness. At the time around diagnosis, they had hoped (and in most cases, prayed) that the child's condition could be cured. This was particularly evident when the child had a congenital degenerative condition, but was currently showing no symptoms. The mothers, whose children had experienced phases of very poor health, relied on their family and friends for emotional support, which was patchy. Occasionally, mothers reported that there were tensions between in-laws:

'We don't have anyone else like that in our family. It must have come from the other side. We don't want to eat in your house. Our children will catch what Munish has'.

Social support and family relationships have been shown to be particularly important for parents with a life-limited child (Mulhern *et al*, 1992; Speechley and Noh, 1992), but parental worry and the distress can result in irritability and tension that, in turn, may reduce the support available from family and friends (Olverholser and Fritz, 1999).

All the mothers cited their children's hospice community team worker as a source of practical and psychological support. Sometimes, 'befrienders' and volunteers from the hospice made a big difference, as did support groups:

'My friend, she came and did the ironing and washed up the pans. I asked her why she did it and she told me she had been thinking how hard it must be, never being able to go to a wedding or a festival time. When we come to the Mothers Group, we talk about our children and we share our thoughts. It makes me have hope in my heart'.

Having a child with a life-limiting illness tears parents' daily lives apart. Often they become overwhelmed with their grief and exhausted through trying to care for their well children, as well as their sick child. Understandably, caring for a life-limited child in such circumstances takes its physical and mental toll on carers and there is a tendency for more visits to doctors and hospitals for their own personal needs (Hatton *et al*, 2004).

'It would be really nice if just once in a while someone could do things for him, so I don't have to feel the strain on my back and shoulders'.

Some studies have focused on the effects of chronic illness on mothers, assuming that they have the largest burden of care (Eiser, 1993). Research is conflicting regarding whether fathers experience more or less distress than mothers when their child is life-limited. Affleck *et al*'s (1991) study of mothers and fathers found that while mothers reported more distress, fathers were reluctant to express their distress outwardly and focused their attention on helping their spouse cope. In our experience, compared with white fathers, South-Asian fathers tended to be more detached from their children's needs.

The outcome of previous research highlighting the stress experienced in families caring for a life-limited child (Brown, 1999, 2001; Chamba *et al*, 1999; Hatton *et al*, 2004) suggests that families from ethnic-minority communities caring for a disabled child may experience greater restrictions on social aspects of their life than white families.

In families where there were other siblings, the life-limited child was almost totally reliant on them for opportunities to play outside school or respite care at the children's hospice. In some families, these young children attended sibling groups at Acorns Children's Hospice. Our experience of working with siblings and their families suggests that in many cases, their daily lives are affected greatly compared with families from other ethnic groups.

Conclusions

Literature about life-limited illness and ethnicity is limited in both its volume and scope. Little is currently known about family roles in paediatric palliative-care settings within different ethnic groups. There is, however, a considerable amount of literature available giving accounts of beliefs about death and funeral rites, focusing on ways of dealing with the body rather than the experience of death and dying within these groups (Firth, 2000; Kalsi, 1996; Brown, 2002). A fundamental weakness of studies to date has been the insensitivity to the processes of change that occur as members of minority ethnic communities adapt to their new societies (Jonker, 1996). Traditional family structures are changing in the UK and often relatives may live too far away for them to be present at the time of death (Firth, 1996). Young South Asians who have been brought up in the UK may not have experienced a death in their family until they themselves are adults.

Diagnosis of a life-limited individual may well be a watershed between two different lifestyles — the pre-diagnostic life, with normal ups and downs; and the post-diagnostic life, where parents feel that their future is unknown and everything is at the mercy of their child's illness. The situation may create confusion and anxiety. Not only do they have to cope with the diagnosis, but they also have to acknowledge that the illness will end in their child's death. Many parents are able vividly to recall the time when they were told that their child was life-limited. They describe their initial reaction as one of extreme shock, a state likened by Goldman (2002) to being similar to that of bereavement.

Over the years, staff at Acorns have cultivated tremendous insights into the experiences, needs and expectations of South-Asian mothers with a life-limited child. This has resulted in the organisation constantly reviewing its policy and practice. Our staff have increased their knowledge, understanding and sensitivity concerning religious and cultural aspects of care. Many of the mothers have been helped to identify strengths that have been previously unnoticed by themselves or their families. They have also been encouraged to develop a positive sense of their own identity and strategies for managing the stress they feel. Parents are reassured that when their child reaches the end stage of life, they will receive help and appropriate facilities will be available to them — for example, having a place set aside for worship or meditation, or appropriate facilities to wash their child after death.

How families deal with the diagnosis of a life-limited child varies. Family members are interdependent: anything that affects one member can affect the family as a whole. It is thought that the way families cope with stress before the diagnosis of the illness may play a critical part in how families cope afterwards.

Recognising that a child's illness is entering another phase may plunge families into renewed crisis with heightened emotions, experienced at a time when parents are beginning to understand the meaning of the medical diagnosis for their child. The interaction between hospice care teams in the community and family key workers plays an important role in maintaining sufficient equilibrium for parents to develop strategies for caring for their child, both in their own home and in the hospice during respite care. All this takes place against a background of the number of people with disabilities increasing and severe learning difficulties being greater in some South-Asian communities compared with white communities (Emerson and Hatton, 1999; Kerr, 2001).

Over the past decade, there has not only been an increasing awareness of the importance of professionals listening to the views of patients and their families, but also a corresponding concern about the stereotypes that have been created. Listening to patients and their families is never easy. It challenges both professionals and service providers. It can also be time-consuming and may unintentionally result in policies based on generalisation and simplification

---

Key points of *Chapter 10*

- Health care should be accessible to all users and relevant to the local population. It should be provided in a manner culturally acceptable to users in the community.
- Provision of accessible and appropriate care to patients from ethnic-minority groups has been recognised as a significant service-development priority.
- The number of children requiring palliative care from South-Asian communities is growing and will continue to do so for the foreseeable future. Nevertheless, families form ethnic-minority communities caring for a disabled child may experience greater restrictions in social aspects of life than white families.
- Evidence-based research into the needs of families with a life-limited child in South-Asian communities is very limited.
- At a time when many other children's hospices are having difficulty attracting referrals from minority ethnic groups, the number of families from South-Asian communities using Acorns Children's Hospices is rising.
- The manner in which the diagnosis of their child's life-limiting illness is disclosed to families plays a significant part in how well individual family members adapt.
- How families cope with the diagnosis of their child's life-limiting illness varies. Family members are interdependent, and anything that affects one member can affect the family as a whole.
- A child's life-limiting illness may pass through several stages from diagnosis to end-of-life care. Mothers' coping strategies change at different phases of their child's illness.
- Families may turn to faith to find a reason for why their child is sick. Families may find comfort in their religion.
- Service providers should strive to provide care that is unbiased and unprejudiced.
- The importance of providing culturally appropriate care in the end-of-life stages of a child's illness and after the child's death is reflected in Acorns Children's Hospices' policies and practice.

---

of peoples' needs. An approach that strives to be unbiased, unprejudiced and as honest as possible is essential. At Acorns Children's Hospices, we have an ongoing commitment to providing the best possible care to life-limited children and their families.

The author acknowledges with gratitude the support and help provided by Hardev Notta in the research project described.

References

ACT (1997) *The Development of Children's Palliative Care Services*. The Association for Children with Life-Threatening or Terminal Conditions and their Families and The Royal College of Paediatrics and Child Health, Bristol

ACT (2003) *The Development of Children's Palliative Care Services*. 2nd edn. The Association for Children with Life-Threatening or Terminal Conditions and their Families and The Royal College of Paediatrics and Child Health, Bristol

Affleck G, Tennen H, Rowe J (1991) *Infants in Crisis: How Parents Cope with Newborn Intensive Care and its Aftermath*. Springer, New York

Atkins K, Rollings J (1998) Looking after their own? Family care-giving among Asian and Afro-Caribbean communities. In: Ahmad W, Atkin K (eds) *'Race' and Community Care*. Open University Press, Buckinghamshire

Bradshaw N, Webb B (1997) *Martin House: Research and Education Study*. Martin House and the Department of Health (DoH), London

Brown E (1999) *Loss, Change and Grief — an Educational Perspective*. David Fulton, London

Brown E (2001) *Supporting Children with Post-Traumatic Stress Disorder — a Handbook for Teachers and Professionals*. David Fulton, London

Brown E (2002) *The Death of a Child — Care for the Child, Support for the Family*. Acorns Children's Hospice, Birmingham

Carpenter B (ed) (1997) *Families in Context: Emerging Trends in Family Support and Early Intervention*. David Fulton, London

Chamba R, Ahmad W, Hirst M, Lawton D, Beresford B (1999) *On the Edge: Minority Ethnic Families Caring for a Severely Disabled Child*. The Policy Press, Bristol

Closs A, Norris C (1997) Outlook uncertain: education for children with poor prognosis — reflections on parental wishes on an appropriate curriculum. *Child Care Health Dev* **21**(6): 387–94

Connors C, Stalker K (2003) *The Views and Experiences of Disabled Children and their Siblings: a Positive Outlook.* Jessica Kingsley, London

Department of Health (DoH) (1997) *The New NHS. Modern, Dependable.* DoH, London

DoH (1998) *The Quality Protects Programme. Transforming Children's Services.* (LAC [98] 28). DoH, London

Eiser C (1993) *Growing Up with Chronic Disease: the Impact on Children and their Families.* Jessica Kingsley, London

Emerson E, Hatton C (1999) Future trends in the ethnic composition of British society among British citizens with disabilities. *Tizzard Learn Disabil Rev* **4**: 28–32

Fanos J, Weiner L (1994) Tomorrow's survivors: siblings of immunodeficiency virus-infected children. *Development Behav Paed* **15**: 43–8

Firth S (1996) 'The good death': attitudes of British Hindus. In: Howarth G, Jupp PC (eds) *Contemporary Issues in the Sociology of Death, Dying and Disposal.* Macmillan, Basingstoke

Firth S (2000) Cross-cultural perspectives on bereavement. In: Dickenson D, Johnson M, Samson J (eds) *Contemporary Issues in the Sociology of Death, Dying and Disposal.* Macmillan, Basingstoke

Firth S (2001) *Wider Horizons — Care of the Dying in a Multicultural Society.* National Council for Hospice and Palliative Care Services, London

Goldman A (ed) (2002) *Care of the Dying Child.* Oxford University Press, Oxford

Hatton C, Akram Y, Shah R, Robertson J, Emerson E (2004) *Supporting South Asian Families with a Child with Severe Disabilities.* Jessica Kingsley, London

Hill L (1994) *Care for the Dying Child and their Families.* Chapman and Hall, London

Hill D, Penso D (1995) *Opening Doors: Improving Access to Hospice and Specialist Palliative Care Services by Members of Black and Ethnic Minority Communities.* Occasional Paper 7. National Council for Specialist and Palliative Care Services, London

Hornby G (1994) *Counselling in Childhood Disability: Skills for Working with Parents.* Chapman and Hall, London

Irish DP, Lundquist KS, Nelson VJ (1999) *Ethical Variations in Dying, Death and Grief: Diversity in Universality.* Taylor and Francis, London

Jonker G (1996) The knife's edge: Muslim burial in the dispora. *Mortality* **1**(1): 27–43

Kalsi S (1996) Change and continuity in the funeral rituals of Sikhs in Britain. In: Howarth G, Jupp PC (eds) *Contemporary Issues in the Sociology of Death, Dying and Disposal.* Macmillan, Basingstoke

Kerr G (2001) Assessing the needs of learning disabled young people with additional disabilities. *J Learn Disabil* **5**: 154–7

Mir G, Nocon A, Ahmad W, Jones L (2001) *Learning Difficulties and Ethnicity.* DoH, London

Mulhern RK, Fairclough DL, Smith B, Douglas SM (1992) Maternal depression. *J Paed Psychol* **17**: 313–26

Nash T (1998) *Development of a Model of Care for Children Suffering from Life-Limited Illness and their Families in the South West.* University of Exeter and the DoH

NHS Executive (2000) *The Vital Connection: an Equalities Framework for the NHS.* DoH. London: NHS

Office for National Statistics (ONS) (2003) Census 2001. http://www. statistics.gov.uk/census (accessed October 2005)

Olverholser J, Burt M (1999) The impact of childhood cancer on the family. *J Psychosoc Oncol* **8**: 71–85

Phillips R, Burt M (1999) *Rachel House: an Independent Evaluation — the Views of Children, Young People and Families.* University of Stirling and Children's Hospice Association of Scotland

Quinton D (2004) *Supporting Parents: Messages from Research.* Jessica Kingsley, London

Scottish Office (1997) *The Children (Scotland Act).* The Stationery Office, Edinburgh

Speechley KN, Noh S (1992) Surviving childhood cancer — social support and parents' psychological adjustment. *J Paed Psychol* **17**: 15–31

Tasker M (1998) *How Can I Tell You?* Association for Care and Children's Health, Bethesda MD

UK Parliament (21 July 2004) *Select Committee on Health (Fourth Report) — Palliative Care.* http://www.parliament.uk/parliamentary_committees/ health_committee.cfm

Welsh Office (1998) *Putting Patients First.* The Stationery Office, Cardiff

CHAPTER 11

The transition from paediatric palliative care to adult services

Erica Brown, Karen White

It matters not how long you live, but how well.
Anon

Transfer to adult services as both an ideology and a process reflects the success of medical advancements in the treatment of life-limiting illnesses. The Royal College of Paediatrics and Child Health (RCPCH) states that 'the need for wider scale planning regarding transition is particularly important in those illnesses once considered to be confined to childhood, where modern treatment advances have led to longer term survival into adult life'. The physical, psychological and developmental needs of this age-group are specific and different from those of children or adults. For example, medications such as opiates are administered orally in children rather than subcutaneously, and gastrostomies are much more commonly performed for nutritional purposes in children than in adults.

Timescales for palliative care also vary enormously, from a few days to many years, depending on the spectrum of life-limiting conditions. Therefore, the transition pathway to adult services requires health professionals and parents to identify and recognise that this group needs an initiative whereby it receives holistic care. This should facilitate a coordinated and developmentally appropriate transition and eventual transfer. Transition as a process, however, involves more than just transferring medical notes and the young person to adult services; it should be 'ideally based on the purposeful, planned movement of adolescents and young adults' (Viner and Keane, 1999). In this chapter, transition to adult services will be discussed with examples of relevance to South Asians.

Erica Brown, Karen White

The size of the problem

Statistical evidence reveals that teenage children represent between 26% and 54% of total numbers of children requiring palliative care (Association of Children with Life Threatening and Terminal Illnesses [ACT], 2003). It is estimated that in a population of 10,000 young people, about two people aged between thirteen and twenty-four years will die. With one in ten children currently being born to black and ethnic-minority groups, of which South Asians form a majority, and this proportion projected to rise because of the relatively larger average family sizes in these groups, it is evident that significant numbers of South-Asian young people are likely to need palliative-care services.

ACT estimates that the number of children in the UK requiring symptom-management and daily care is likely to be between 6000 and 10,000, and that this will increase as therapies continue to evolve.

Main categories of conditions requiring palliative care in children and young adults

Some of the conditions requiring palliative-care provision are congenital (eg. microcephaly), others genetic (eg. tyrosinaemia) or acquired (eg. leukaemia). Others manifest themselves and are diagnosed in adolescence and young adulthood. The RCPCH and ACT's *Palliative Care Service Guidelines* (2003) describe four main categories of condition (*Panel 11.1*) of which the last three non-cancerous groups are currently more common among South Asians.

Decision-making by children and young adults

In England, Wales and Northern Ireland, once young persons reach eighteen years of age, provided they have the capacity to think and decide independently, decisions around their health care rest solely with them. Young people between sixteen and eighteen years may also have the capacity to judge and to understand for themselves under the Family Law Act (1969). However, until 1986, the right of children under sixteen years of age to make their own decisions about their medical care did not exist. Cooper (1999) refers to a 'protectionist philosophy' underpinning childcare that views young people as fragile, incompetent,

---

Panel 11.1: Trajectories of palliative care in young people

- Life-threatening conditions for which curative treatment may be feasible, but can fail. Palliative care may be necessary during periods of prognostic uncertainty and when treatment is unsuccessful. Young people in long-term remission or following successful curative treatment are not included. Examples include cancer and organ failure of heart, liver or kidneys.
- Conditions where there may be long periods of intensive treatment aimed at prolonging life and allowing participation in normal activities, but premature death is still possible or inevitable. Examples include cystic fibrosis, Duchenne Muscular Dystrophy and HIV/AIDS.
- Progressive conditions without curative treatment options, where treatment is exclusively palliative and may commonly extend over many years. Examples include Batten disease, muscopolysaccharidosis and variant Creutzfeldt-Jakob disease (CJD).
- Severe neurological disability, which may cause weakness and susceptibility to health complications. Deterioration may be unpredictable, but is not usually progressive. Examples include severe multiple disabilities following brain or spinal-cord injuries, and severe cerebral palsy.

---

powerless, and unable to care for themselves. The same author believes that this may result in young people being denied a right to be involved in their own care. Although young people under the age of sixteen years have no statutory rights, they can be 'Gillick competent' if they are able to demonstrate an understanding of the issues involved (1985). Therefore, medical professionals are required to judge the competence of the young persons and then to involve them in decisions made on their behalf. (In Scotland, young people aged sixteen years and over are presumed to be competent to make decisions.)

The plan for transition to adult services is an important one. Where health professionals have been involved in the care of the young person before transition, they should attend the young person's multidisciplinary review, which typically occurs at fourteen years of age, and advise on services that are likely to be required. The young person's health records should be transferred to adult services with consent of the child if possible, and, if necessary, from the parents.

Little has been written about the participation of life-limited young people in decisions concerning their care. Collaborative partnership extends beyond the relationship between the parents and the health professional to one that encourages the young persons to be involved in decisions that are made on their behalf. Riley (1996) and ACT (2003) believe that all people should be able to voice their opinions, a view underpinned by the Children Act (1989) which states: 'children must be kept informed about what happens to them and

---

Panel 11.2: Critical elements of transitional care

- Comprehensive written information about the adult unit at an early stage.
- Combined paediatric and adult clinics with the opportunity for young people to discuss and sample new facilities and staff, accompanied by a paediatric team member.
- Joint visits to the young person by paediatric and adult nurses.
- Consideration of the young person's emotional well-being post transfer.

Panel 11.3: Reasons why transitional care is often inadequate

- Families may have developed a strong attachment to paediatric services over many years and resist transfer to a specialist consultant they do not know.
- Consultant paediatricians may develop a strong relationship with families and be reluctant to hand over care.
- Parents fear that adult services will be less comprehensive and less personal.
- Parents fear that adult services will be less well coordinated.
- Equivalent adult services may not exist.
- Families may fear that they will be unsupported in the terminal phase of their child's care, especially if this coincides with transition.
- The assessment of young person's holistic needs (including their emotional readiness for transition) may have been neglected.

---

participate when decisions are made about their future'.

Despite this recommendation, young people are not always given opportunities that enable them to make their views known. It may be that a potential exists for young person's autonomy to be overlooked under the umbrella of family-centred care because the focus is often on parents making decisions on behalf of their child; indeed, parents need support and encouragement to enable their son or daughter to develop as much autonomy as possible.

Although women usually take the main responsibility for looking after children with life-limiting illnesses in South-Asian households, decisions are often made by the men folk, usually elders of the family, and therefore legal and ethical factors relating to confidentiality, consent and refusal of treatment can become major issues for this group of young people. However, with good support, guidance and understanding from health professionals, these important family ties and interactions can often prove positive in the long-term care of these children.

Critical elements of the transition process

Critical elements suggested by Powncenby (1996) in the transition process are shown in *Panel 11.2.*

ACT (2001) identified seven reasons why the transition process from paediatric services to adult services is inadequate (*Panel 11.3*).

For many young South Asians with a life-limiting illness, their families provide the bulk of their care, typically with an array of support services that may include primary care teams, community paediatricians, occupational therapists and nursing teams such as Diana Teams (funded by the Diana Princess of Wales Memorial Fund to support children with cancer), working collaboratively with social workers overseen by a community paediatrician. In some regions, multiagency children's palliative-care groups also exist, providing care and support for young people up to the age of nineteen years. These primary care teams may not have adequate knowledge of life-limiting conditions such as metabolic disorders and progressive degenerative illnesses, which are particularly common in the Muslim community, where there is a high incidence of consanguineous marriages. Often there is a paucity of appropriate respite care for this group, with palliative-care services focusing largely, albeit inadequately, on elderly South-Asian patients with cancer.

Adolescents

In 2001, the ACT/RCPCH Working Party made a plea for flexible provision matched to the needs of young people (aged thirteen to twenty-four years). In line with this, some children's hospices have evolved services to care for children up to nineteen years of age. Respite care is one of the hallmarks of this need, and although children's hospices such as Martin House (Wetherby, West Yorkshire), Douglas House (Oxford) and Acorns (Birmingham) have expanded care to provide for the needs of adolescents and young adults, there is a huge gap in the provision of care outside the home for this age-group.

Recognition of the specific and often subtle changes associated with the period of adolescence is almost universal. Adolescence is a time of immense change — physical, mental, psychological, spiritual and social. The adolescent faces new and previously uncharted ground, such as employment, body image, sexuality and personal identity. Furthermore, the transition towards adulthood is a pathway that all of society expects adolescents to tread. Understanding the rapid changes in relation to the physical, social, emotional and cognitive development of young South Asians is pivotal in matching the care to the needs of young people with life-limiting illnesses.

Adolescence is a journey of discovery, turmoil, challenges, experimentations, ambivalence, egocentricity, confidence and self-doubt, combined with unfolding changes physically, emotionally and intellectually (Cooper, 1999). Coping with a life-threatening illness is therefore a monumental undertaking. Unlike young children, adolescents generally perceive death as irreversible. Therefore acceptance of personal death is particularly difficult because for many young people their lives are orientated towards a future. It should be remembered, however, that many of the anxieties that life-limited adolescents encounter have their roots firmly embedded in youth culture, which accentuates differences between life-limited young people and their non-life-limited peers.

Several studies have attempted to define the developmental stages of adolescence, dividing the transitional period from childhood to young adulthood into three phases: early, middle and late. Some adolescents in the late phase may be almost completely dependent on their parents for their care at a time when chronic and progressive illness reaches a crisis.

The societal perception of adolescence and adult status varies between cultures. In Western society, there is no accepted age that defines adult status in all aspects of life. For example, a young person may marry at sixteen years, hold a driving licence at seventeen years, and vote at eighteen years. By contrast, in South-Asian cultures, adolescents have adult responsibility early. For example, many girls learn to cook and do the housework from an age as early as twelve years. It is therefore important to be mindful of the developmental stages that South-Asian adolescents assume (*Panel 11.4*).

Panel 11.4: Developmental objectives for South-Asian adolescents

- learning about religion and the scriptures
- taking adult responsibility early in their lives
- developing a set of their own values and morals
- personal and peer-group identity — in a community setting
- changes in the perception of body image
- developing career pathways
- forming autonomy financially and socially.

Adolescents are often very knowledgeable about their illness and their prognosis, and the effects these have on those that care for them. Some will need to explore 'reasons' for their life-limiting illness (Hart and Schneider, 1997) and in particular why they have to endure physical and cognitive deterioration. Having a life-limiting illness can be exceptionally isolating and many young people lose contact with their peer group outside a palliative-care or special-needs setting. Here, parents and the extended family members come into their own in providing religious and spiritual support for the life-limited child. The child or adolescent may be shielded from the outside world, as some South-Asian families would not want knowledge of their child's illness to become public as this may affect the marriage prospects of other children in the family.

Many young people with life-limiting illnesses will require extensive support from a range of agencies up to and including the end-of-life stage of their care. Support is often viewed as incompatible with adult status and inconsistent with autonomy. Furthermore, young people may experience agencies as intrusive and controlling. True support enables personal autonomy and self-sufficiency, encouraging young people to choose how and when they use the services available to them. Many South-Asian families are not aware of the various support options during this difficult transition time; *Panel 11.5* highlights some of them.

Panel 11.5: Support services available to young people with life-limiting conditions

- **The Connexions Service** — for thirteen to nineteen year-olds. Personal advisers link in with specialist support services. They are supported by a comprehensive service delivery structure with local organisations working together within Connexions Partnerships.
- **Learning and Skills Council** — responsible for the development, planning, funding and management of all post-sixteen-years education and learning (except higher education) and work-based training for young people. The Council has a statutory duty to take account of assessments arranged by the Connexions Service.
- **Strategic Health Authority** — should agree with primary care groups and trusts how the local health authority can meet the individual needs of young people. Health authorities and trusts should also inform young people and their carers about voluntary organisations that might provide support.

Meeting the transitional needs of young people with life-limited illnesses requires flexible working on the part of statutory agencies. They need to communicate and agree policies and protocols that work towards providing a 'seamless' service. The objective should be to provide integrated, high-quality holistic support, focused on the needs of the young person and their family. Such provision should be based on a shared perspective and should build, whenever possible, on mutual understanding and agreement. Services should adopt a client-centred approach to the delivery of care to ensure the changing needs and priorities of each young person. However, comprehensive, coordinated, inter-agency planning is probably the exception rather than the rule in most cases.

Education

Education is an entitlement for young people under the age of nineteen years and plays a major part in preparing young people for the transition to adulthood. Although more and more South-Asian mothers speak English, children may have been looked after by grandparents who are more likely to be non-English speakers, which may affect the level of communication in English achieved by the young person, particularly where they experience a learning difficulty. Current provision in further education has been shaped by attitudes and political policies in recent years. The document *Young Adults' Transition Project – Optimum Health Services* (NHS, 1999) highlighted that the time of transition for young people with special needs was particularly difficult. Furthermore, the Beattie report, *Implementing Inclusiveness: Realising Potential* (Beattie, 1999) concluded that 'young people with learning disabilities are at risk of social exclusion and difficult transition on leaving school and subsequent transitions'.

According to the Disability Discrimination Act (1995), Section 1(1), a person has a disability if they 'have a physical or mental impairment which has a substantial and long-term adverse effect on their ability to carry out normal day-to-day activities'. Most young people with life-limiting conditions will have a Statement of Special Educational Needs that outlines their individual needs and the measures that must be taken to meet those needs. The *Special Educational Needs Code of Practice* (2001) outlines several principles that underpin transition and transition planning, taking into account the requirements of a young person and their family. The transition process should be participative, holistic, supportive, evolving, inclusive and collaborative.

All young people with a Statement of Special Educational Needs should, in law, have the Statement reviewed annually. Some young people will remain in school until they are nineteen years of age. In the final year of their schooling, the Connexions Service has a responsibility (under Section 140 of the Learning and Skills Act [2000]) to coordinate transition from school to the continuing education sector and for assessing Social Services support. Where a placement in a specialist college is appropriate for a young person, a copy of the student's Transition Plan should be sent to the local Learning and Skills Council.

For any young person, a course at college or university necessitates a period of transition. For young people with life-limiting illnesses, this transition marks a significant and important part in their lives as they move from a childhood role to adult status. The major role of further education is to enable young people to make best use of this transition, offering them the educational and vocational opportunities to which they have a right. Opportunities will vary from location to location, but an increasing number of colleges now make education available to a wide range of students, sometimes in conjunction with social or health services or voluntary organisations.

Further education should aim to meet individual student needs through offering a tailored educational programme that is constructed within a curriculum framework, using age and ability-appropriate activities, language, resources and teaching strategies. Technological support may be an important component in individual student learning. Part-time courses may sometimes be delivered through outreach services.

Vocational guidance is an important part of the Transition Plan and the Connexions Service should assist the young person and their parents to access the most appropriate provision, providing counselling and support as appropriate. Where the young person concerned requires services from the local authority after leaving school, this should be arranged with multi-agency support including the provision of further education. Some young people may become independent of their families, moving into higher education and pursuing other personal goals. Assessment of each person's needs is a unique process, which should be incorporated into a plan of action that can be developed.

A very limited number of young people will achieve independent living, provided they are given adequate assistance in moving away from home. In this regard, some studies have shown that South Asians with chronic health needs or disabilities are likely to be disadvantaged in terms of paid employment, housing and income (Chamba *et al*, 1999; Hatton *et al*, 2004). In the case of young people who use the services of children's hospice care, whether this is community-based or hospice-based, there are very few equitable services available once they have reached the age of nineteen years.

Many adult palliative-care services are for elderly people with cancer. The exception is the newly opened service at Douglas House in Oxford, UK, for young adults aged eighteen-to-forty years. However, as yet it is too early to evaluate how service-users view the support they receive and whether it helps them develop strategies for 'continuing to make their mark' in a way that encourages them to gain a sense of purpose and meaning in the time they have left. Our enquiries suggest that, to date, there are very few South-Asian patients using this service (Brown, 2004).

Examples of transitional journeys

To illustrate some of the issues that life-limited young people may have in accomplishing adolescent objectives and how these may impact on the transitional journey, a few examples are given in *Panels 11.6–11.8*. Client names have been changed to protect anonymity and do not refer to clients at Acorns Hospices.

Panel 11.6: Examples of transitional journeys — Munisha

Munisha is a fifteen-year-old Hindu girl who had thalassaemia major. She has had two unsuccessful bone transplants and received courses of immonusuppressive therapy and is currently receiving palliative care. She is aware of her diagnosis and has been kept fully informed. She has lost contact with many of her peers and has decided not to sit her examinations. A couple of her close friends still visit her at home once a week, but they are busy revising for their exams. She is delayed in puberty, has alopecia and is very underweight and short for her age.

Treatment can sometimes result in physical changes to the young person that may cause stress and poor body-image — at a time when self-esteem and a positive body-image may be crucial. The loss of Munisha's hair (*Panel 11.6*) may signify loss of her femininity, as may her weight loss. Her hair loss may well leave her with feelings of gross disfigurement and difficulties in the context of her already altered physique. It may also be a factor in why she doesn't want to continue with her studies or see many of her friends. She is likely to be isolated and withdrawn. She will fully comprehend her prognosis (as may her peers), but actually talking about her wishes and needs may be incredibly difficult. She has previously experienced life without a life-limited illness. She is becoming increasingly dependent on her parents physically, emotionally and even financially. Her independence, self-image and personal role in her community have changed dramatically. Munisha's parents may 'wrap her in cotton wool' in an attempt to protect her and extend her life. Her sexual identity will undoubtedly change and her realisation of the loss of future hopes and goals may also contribute to a real sense of despair.

Duchenne muscular dystrophy affects boys and is an inherited condition (mothers are the carrier). Boys are usually in an electric wheelchair by their early teens. Young people affected by this condition will experience a gradual loss of their motor skills over a period of years. They will have seen their peers and siblings undertaking the tasks of adolescence and will inevitably need support when attempting to perform these same tasks. Many Duchenne muscular dystrophy sufferers will have lived with the knowledge that their condition means they will die during their adolescence. As they grow older, the realisation that they will probably not experience a sexual relationship, have children, or follow their career path of choice, may result in despair and depression. By the very nature of their condition, these young people will not have been able to achieve independence — physically, emotionally or socially. In turn, the amount of privacy they receive, or indeed have expectations of, will differ greatly compared with their non-life-limited peers.

In this particular case, Hasan (*Panel 11.7*) may feel a real sense of anger

---

Panel 11.7: Examples of transitional journeys — Hassan

Hasan is a seventeen-year-old Muslim boy who suffers from the progressive muscular degenerative disorder, Duchenne Muscular Dystrophy. He is unable to walk and uses an electric wheelchair. He has limited upper-body movement and is completely dependent on his mother for all aspects of his personal care. He has very mild learning difficulties and attends mainstream college. His communication skills are very good. Hasan's best friend has invited him to attend his eighteenth birthday party, which is being held at a wheelchair-friendly venue in the next town. Hasan has asked his parents if he can attend the party, and if his mother will take him. Unfortunately, Hasan's father feels that he needs the use of the family's only mode of transport, the adapted car, to attend a family wedding, to which Hasan will not be taken.

---

towards his parents for using the vehicle that has been specifically adapted for his use. However, how can Hasan display anger towards his parents when he is totally dependent on them for all of his care needs? He cannot 'storm out' of the house, 'bang' doors or 'take himself off' for a few hours to calm down. He is left with pent-up anger and emotions. However, the family's predicament can also be understood; they do not want to 'advertise' his disability to the hundreds who would be attending the wedding, perhaps because of fear of the wider impact on other family members, such as marriage prospects of another sibling.

The next case study highlights the difficulties of those adolescents who are unable to communicate their needs. Gurjeet (*Panel 11.8*) is able to communicate non-verbally by using gesture and eye-contact. Occasionally, she uses an electric speaking machine. She watches television and sees how people of her own age are leading their lives and how this differs vastly from her own experience. The clothes that she wears, the music that she listens to, and the bedtime and personal care she receives may also be aimed at a much younger person than herself. This may result in frustration, anger and withdrawal. Physiologically, Gurjeet will have undergone the same hormonal and bodily changes as any young woman.

Before the progression of her disease, Gurjeet may have had distinct career

---

Panel 11.8: Examples of transitional journeys — Gurjeet

Gurjeet is a nineteen-year-old Sikh girl with childhood-onset leukodystrophy. She is often agitated, suffers from involuntary movements, and has difficulties with feeding, which requires a gastrostomy. She is at home most of the week, as there are no suitable education or respite facilities available locally. Her grandmother, who does not speak English, is her main carer.

---

aspirations. These career goals will have been scuppered by her physical disability, limited communication skills and lack of accessible resources. Another consideration is Gurjeet's own expectations for her future, as well as those of parents and professionals, who may well be unable to comprehend that she has young adult aspirations and hopes. Gurjeet's understanding of English may be rudimentary in view of her learning disability and the inability of her main carer to speak in English.

These case studies illustrate the real and visible differences that life-limited South-Asian adolescents encounter when journeying through the period of transition towards adulthood. During this time, young people usually strive to achieve emancipation from their parents. Shopping trips, cinema visits as well as a reluctance to participate in family gatherings are just some of the ways of seeking freedom from parents, although for the South-Asian child, it is unusual to be left out of family events. Disagreements and debates around politics, religion and the pop culture of the day may become commonplace as young people become more questioning and begin to develop their own morals and values.

For young people suffering with a life-limiting condition, the tasks that most of us take for granted become incredibly difficult, if not near-impossible to achieve. Hasan is never likely to leave home and become physically and financially independent, and Munisha may experience resistance from her parents if she strives to be autonomous. She will inevitably be inhibited by the progression of the disease. Gurjeet's limited communication skills may prevent her from informing carers or professionals of her fears, anxieties or indeed the pain that she may be suffering. These three young people all have to face a future, no matter how short. It is a very different future from the one they would like, and which society expects.

Conclusions

Concerns about the transition of young people with life-limiting conditions from paediatric to adult care were first highlighted by ACT in the 2001 report, *Palliative Care for Young People Aged 13 to 24 Years*. The document stated: 'for rare disorders, especially degenerative conditions... where young people have outlived their predicted life expectancy, there is no equivalent service to transfer them to'. If this is the case nationally, what hope do South-Asian children with life-limiting conditions have?

More recently the Royal College of Nursing (RCN) document *Adolescent Transition Care* (2004) highlighted four potential areas of difficulty when planning adult provision for young people:

- lack of specialist knowledge in adult teams and lack of confidence in knowledge
- lack of specific service provision for young people
- lack of understanding and appreciation of young people's needs and issues in both paediatric and adult healthcare sectors
- professional attitudes.

Within the health service, there are still no regulations for managing the transition of young life-limited people to adult care settings, although the Government's Select Committee Inquiry into Palliative Care recommendations (July, 2004) makes a call for the overview of service provision.

Introduction of cultural-diversity issues that pervade postgraduate and

---

Key points of *Chapter 11*

- Young people should be intimately involved in choices and decision-making at every level.
- Confidentiality should be respected and upheld at all times.
- Flexibility and anticipation of young people's needs should be integral to care at times of transition from children's services to adult services and at end-of-life care.
- Continuity of support should be provided at times of transition.
- Tension between the dependency and inter-dependency of young people should be acknowledged.
- Families should be included in care plans (in consultation with the young person).
- Young people who have partners should be enabled to include them in choices regarding care (if the young person wishes).
- Psychological, spiritual and cultural aspects of care should be integral to service provision.
- Care packages acknowledging cultural issues should be reviewed frequently.
- Equipment and mobility aids should be regularly updated and matched to the individual needs of the young person.
- Personal relationships should be encouraged and incorporated into care plans (but not, for South Asians, sexual experiences, since these would be against their culture and religion).
- Peer-group activities should be encouraged and provision made to enable these to happen.
- The environment in which young people are cared for should be age-appropriate.

Based on ACT (2001).

---

undergraduate courses of both doctors and nurses will go a long way to improving the plight of South Asians who it is feared will otherwise be sidelined. Service providers have a duty to help young people from all cultures, understand what is available to them and how to access the support available. They should also have a commitment towards working collaboratively with other agencies on a regular basis, rather than on a crisis basis, and should be suitably experienced and qualified to work with young people and their families. Understanding generic adolescence issues such as relationships, independent living and leisure interests, in addition to the specific needs of young South-Asian people with life-limiting illnesses, will contribute enormously in planning transition from paediatric services to adult care. All this is likely to result in positive outcomes, irrespective of the prognosis for the young people concerned.

References

ACT/National Council for Hospice and Palliative Care Services/Scottish Partnership Agency for Palliative Care and Cancer Care (2001) *Palliative Care for Young People 13–24*. ACT, Bristol

ACT/RCPCH (1997) *A Guide to the Development of Children's Palliative Care Services*. The Association for Children with Life-Threatening or Terminal Conditions and their Families/Royal College of Paediatricians and Child Health, Bristol

ACT/RCPCH (2003) *A Guide to the Development of Children's Palliative Care Services*. 2nd edn. The Association for Children with Life-Threatening or Terminal Conditions and their Families/Royal College of Paediatricians and Child Health, Bristol

Beattie R (1999) *Implementing Inclusiveness: Realising Potential*. Scottish Executive Report, Edinburgh

British Medical Association (2000) *Consent, Rights and Choices in Health Care for Children and Young People*. BMA, London

Brown E (2004) Personal communication

Chamba R, Ahmad W, Hirst M, Lawton D, Beresford B (1999) *On the Edge: Minority Ethnic Families Caring for a Severely Disabled Child*. The Policy Press, Bristol

Cooper C (1999) *Continuing Care of Sick Children: Examining the Impact of Chronic Illness*. Quay Books, Salisbury

Department for Education and Skills (DfES) (2001) *The Special Educational Needs Code of Practice*. DfES, Nottingham

Department of Health (DoH) (1991) *The Children Act and Regulations. Vol 6. Children with Disabilities.* HMSO, London

Department of Health (DoH)/Department for Education and Employment and the Home Office (2000) *Framework for the Assessment of Children in Need and their Families.* The Stationery Office, London

Gillick v West Norfolk and Wisbeach Health Authority (1985) (3 AII ER 402 HL)

Hart D, Schneider D (1997) Spiritual care for children with cancer. *Semin Oncol* **13**(4): 263–70

Hatton C, Akram Y, Shah R, Robertson J, Emerson E (2004) *Supporting South Asian Families with a Child with Severe Disabilities.* Jessica Kingsley, London

NHS (1999) *Young Adults' Transition Project — Optimum Health Services.* NHS, London

Powncenby J (1996) *The Coming of Age Project — A Study of the Transition from Paediatric to Adult Care and Treatment Adherence among Young People with Cystic Fibrosis.* Cystic Fibrosis Trust, London

Riley R (1996) Children as customers too. *Br J Community Nurs* **1**: 158–9

Royal College of Nursing (RCN) (2004) *Adolescent Transition Care — Guidance for Nursing Staff.* RCN, London

UK Government (1969) The Family Law Reform Act. HMSO, London

UK Government (1995) Disability Discrimination Act. HMSO, London

UK Government (2000) The Learning and Skills Act. HMSO, London

UK Parliament (21 July, 2004) *Select Committee on Health. 4th Report. Palliative Care*

Viner R, Keane M (1998) *Youth Matters: Evidence-based Best Practice for the Care of Young People in Hospital: Caring for Children in Health Services.* Action for Sick Children, London

CHAPTER 12

Reflections of a Macmillan nurse

Glenys Mitchell

The beginning of wisdom is being able to say 'I don't know'.
  Anon

In this chapter, I aim to show how Western stereotypes can affect the care of a patient with a different world-view. In doing so, I shall use an example of pain and its management in a patient, which on reflection I should have dealt with differently. One of the principal functions of palliative medicine is the prevention and control of distressing symptoms, of which the most common is pain. The relief of pain is one of the most effective expressions of the ethical principle of beneficence. By preventing the occurrence and controlling the intensity of this symptom, the palliative-care team is fulfilling one of its highest ethical duties (Wilkinson, 1995).

The limited empirical evidence available suggests that perceptions and expressions of pain are strongly shaped by culture. The exact location and meaning of pain has to be ascertained accurately, as a South-Asian patient may say that his 'heart is burning' or 'hurting', meaning in fact that he is upset.

Reasons cited for the inadequate management of cancer pain are knowledge deficits and inappropriate attitudes about cancer pain, particularly regarding the use of opioids (Elliot, 1992; Cleeland *et al*, 1986). In 1994, the UK General Medical Council (UK GMC) recommended that medical undergraduate education incorporate palliative care pain-management into their curricula (GMC, 1994).

Glenys Mitchell

What is reflective practice?

The principle that health professionals should become reflective practitioners is now commonly acknowledged, and is increasingly being realised. The essential purpose of reflective practice is to enable the practitioner to access, understand and learn through their lived experiences and, as a consequence, take congruent action towards developing increasing effectiveness within the context of what is understood as desirable practice (Johns, 1995). Reflective practice is one way to use experience to promote personal and professional growth. Examining and analysing events that have affected patients can help nurses gain a better understanding of their actions and feelings, which can in turn lead them to question theories and practices. Integrating new knowledge with increased self-awareness can help their practice in future to promote effective, individualised care (Stewart, 2003).

A case study: Mrs N

To illustrate the importance of reflective practice, I will use John's model of structured reflection (Johns and Freshwater, 1998) as a framework.

Mrs N, a seventy-three year-old Muslim South Asian woman was referred to me for symptom-management during her hospital stay. She had been diagnosed with oesophageal cancer several months earlier, and had undergone radiotherapy treatment, which had sadly proved ineffective. She was now in the end-stage of her disease and was showing considerable distress when I came to see her. Prior to being referred to me, she had been prescribed fentanyl transdermal (opioid) patches for her pain and over time the dose had reached 150µg/hour over seventy-two hours. Fentanyl is an opioid analgesic and is most useful in patients with stable, chronic, intractable cancer-related pain for whom the oral route of administration is no longer an option (Twycross *et al*, 2002).

For some unspecified reason, the fentanyl patch had been discontinued a few days prior to referral to me and an alternative opioid, diamorphine 20mgs/24hrs via a syringe driver, had been started in its place. A fentanyl 150µg patch is equivalent to 160mgs diamorphine in twenty-four hours (Dept of Medicines Management, 1997), so it was no surprise to me that Mrs N was in severe distress from her pain.

Mrs N did not speak English. As her son was present and because she was in severe distress, I assessed the situation using her son as an interpreter, although this can have its disadvantages as family members may be deliberately selective in their translation so as not to alarm a patient (Spruyt, 1999). Because she was a frail old lady, and because it was difficult to assess accurately exactly how much of her distress was caused by pain and how much was fear and anxiety, I decided to proceed cautiously with increasing her analgesia. I suggested diamorphine 40mgs/24hrs via the syringe driver; I also suggested adding levomepromazine 12.5mg/24hrs via the same syringe driver. This would provide both an anti-emetic and a mild sedative, which would be beneficial in reducing her anxiety and restlessness (BNF, 2003).

The intention behind 'sedation' is good — to relieve distress, but not to bring about the patient's death. Intractable symptoms are a source of major distress for patients, families and professionals, and it seems entirely justified that a slight risk of shortening life is outweighed by helping an individual achieve a peaceful death. This is sometimes referred to as the doctrine of double effect and has traditionally been associated with use of morphine (Thorns, 2002).

I explained the management plan to Mrs N's son and ensured that he understood and was amenable to this course of action. Although I could not directly speak with Mrs N, due to the language barrier, I felt that I was fulfilling my duty of care by offering safe and competent care to her. However, by accepting the consent of her son rather than hers, it is possible that I was not respecting her autonomy (NMC, 2002).

When I came to see her the next day, she appeared to be pain free and was sleeping peacefully. I continued to visit her daily to monitor her condition and a few days later her son expressed his concern that she was sleeping all the time; he would prefer that the sedation was reduced to enable her to talk to her family. I explained to him that there was often a fine balance between keeping the symptoms under control and ensuring that there was minimal sedation. However, he was quite insistent so I agreed to reduce the dose of levomepromazine by half to 6.25mgs/24hrs. This is considered to be a dose that would not normally cause sedation (BNF, 2003).

When I visited the next day, the dose had been reduced but she was still sleeping most of the time. Whilst I was there, the nursing staff came to attend to her and I heard her crying out as they changed her position. They reported that she was complaining of pain on movement, so I suggested increasing the diamorphine to 50mgs/24hrs, which was done. A day later, I received a phone call from another one of Mrs N's sons, requesting that the increased medication be reduced because she was not able to talk to her family. I attempted to explain that she needed that amount because she was experiencing pain on movement. He was, however, very insistent too and requested that I come to the ward and speak to his brother, who was with Mrs N. When I came on to the ward, I discovered that the family had also approached the doctors, who had already reduced the diamorphine to 40mgs/24hrs.

I felt quite angry towards the family because, in my opinion, they seemed more interested in their own needs above their mother's comfort, and I felt anger towards the medical staff for (as I saw it) giving in to the family's demands.

Mrs N's condition generally remained fairly stable and she was comfortable most of the time. The ward staff reported that there were occasions when she experienced pain, particularly when she was moved. Her son, who usually stayed with her when I visited, told me that his mother was now able to converse with her family and he appeared to be satisfied with the situation. She died a few days later.

I was subsequently quite troubled over this incident. For no apparent reason, I was questioning my actions in managing Mrs N. Although I was confident that my clinical judgement was sound, and the doses of medications given were correct and adequate, I felt uncomfortable with my interaction and quite a deep sense of failure that I may not have acted as Mrs N's advocate (NMC, 2002). It was then that I realised that I had been attempting to treat Mrs N from a Western perspective of palliative care, which prioritises pain relief, and I had not necessarily been receptive to the cues her South-Asian family was giving me.

The process of reflection

According to Gatrad and Sheikh (2002), an extended family structure is typical of the Muslim community and family dynamics are often very different from those customary in Western society. Families are often hierarchical and patriarchal, and palliative care should be delivered to these families in a way that acknowledges these factors.

A major difference between British and South-Asian cultures relates to the concept of 'family' versus 'self'. Decision-making amongst the South Asians is not the sole domain of the patient, as in the autonomous Euro-American model, but is heavily influenced by family dynamics and is more of a patriarchal model (Boyle, 1998). In the South-Asian model, Boyle suggests that because of the many intrinsic (family-centred) and extrinsic (environment-, professional- and care giver-related) variables that influence perception of pain and its relief, an 'aversive milieu' is created by the situation in which the family, patient and the nurse all find that they are not satisfied with the effort of managing symptoms.

Gatrad and Sheikh (2002) say that undue suffering has no place in Islam and if death is hastened in the process of giving adequate analgesia, then there is no objection to this form of symptom-management. They go on to add that it is important to notify relatives that if opioids are used to control pain, these may have a negative impact on cognitive ability and levels of consciousness; therefore, the use of this group of drugs may affect a patient's ability to reaffirm his or her declaration of faith, the Shahadah (see *Chapter 4*), before death.

As I reflected on this, I began to realise that my lack of knowledge and understanding of the Muslim faith and culture had contributed in creating a difficult situation which led to my feelings of anger and frustration. Murphy and Clark (1993) state that nursing research has revealed that nurses experience frustration from not understanding their 'ethnic' patients' cultures, and Lea (1994) supports this by adding that nurses need to understand their patients from their cultural perspective if they are to provide culturally sensitive care.

My prior knowledge of any ethnic-minority culture was, I have to confess, quite limited, largely stereotypical and anecdotal. Mattson and Johnson (1992) suggest that nurses must discover how their values and attitudes influence their perceptions of patients and their nursing care. Such awareness would also help them avoid feeling threatened by conflicts of values, and enable them to respond rationally and non-judgementally when confronted with other cultural norms.

Neuberger (1995) argues that the desire to put those who are different from oneself into categories leads to depersonalisation. The individual concerned will usually be pleased to explain something of the nature of his or her religious beliefs and cultural traditions to a healthcare professional. This interaction can impart valuable information to the carer and promote the development of a deeper relationship between the patient (or relative) and the carer. It also provides an excellent opportunity for all to learn about each others' different traditions and cultures.

Conclusion

Reflecting on this episode has enabled me to examine and critically analyse some of my assumptions, values and attitudes about the delivery of palliative care — not only to ethnic-minority patients and their families, but also to patients and families of any ethnic or cultural background. In future, I will endeavour to improve my interactions with patients and their families by attempting to forge a trusting and mutually respectful relationship with them. It seems that asking pertinent questions to elicit their needs and concerns, and to gain as much information as possible to provide the care to which they are entitled, may be the wisest strategy.

> ### Key points of *Chapter 12*
>
> - Reflective practice enables the practitioner to access, understand and learn through lived experiences.
> - Perceptions and expressions of pain are strongly shaped by culture.
> - Decision-making amongst South Asians is often a patriarchal model that is heavily influenced by family dynamics.
> - Identify one relative for regular communication.
> - Using heavy analgesia without first discussing it with family members may create anxiety and anger if last rites cannot be carried out as a result.

References

Cleeland CS, Cleeland LM, Dar R, Rinehardt LC (1986) Factors influencing physician management of cancer pain. *Cancer* **58**: 796–800

Department of Medicines Management (1997) *Guidelines for the Use of Drugs in Symptom Control.* Keele University, Keele

Elliot TE, Elliot BA (1992) Physicians' attitudes and beliefs about the use of morphine for cancer pain. *J Pain Symptom Manage* **7**: 141–8

Gatrad AR, Sheikh A (2002) Palliative care for Muslims. *Int J Palliat Nurs* **8**(11): 526–31

General Medical Council (GMC) (1993) *Tomorrow's Doctors: Recommendation on Undergraduate Medical Education.* GMC, London

Johns C (1995) Framing learning through reflection within carpers fundamental ways of knowing in nursing. *J Adv Nurs* **22**: 226–34

Johns C, Freshwater D (1998) *Transforming Nursing through Reflective Practice.* Blackwell Science, Oxford

Lea A (1994) Nursing in today's multicultural society: a transcultural perspective. *J Adv Nurs* **20**: 307–13

Mattson S, Johnson L (1992) Integration of cultural content into a psychiatric nursing course to change students' attitudes and decrease anxiety. *Nurse Educ* **17**(4): 5

Murphy K, Clark JM (1993) Nurses' experiences of caring for ethnic minority clients. *J Adv Nurs* **18**: 442–50

Neuberger J (1995) Cultural issues in palliative care. In: Doyle D, Hanks GWC, Macdonald N (eds) *Oxford Textbook of Palliative Medicine.* Oxford University Press, Oxford

Nursing and Midwifery Council (NMC) (2002) *Code of Professional Conduct.*

NMC Publications, London

Pitches D (2000) *Health Services in Birmingham for Black and Minority Ethnic Older People: Report of a Baseline Survey for Birmingham.* Race Action Partnership. Birmingham Health Authority, Birmingham

Royal Pharmaceutical Society of Great Britain (2003) *British National Formulary.* British Medical Association (BMA), London

Spruyt O (1999) Community-based palliative care for Bangladeshi patients in East London: accounts of bereaved carers. *Palliat Med* **13**(2): 119–30

Stewart M (2003) Reflecting on the psychosocial care of patients with a terminal illness. *Prof Nurse* **18**(7): 402–5

Thorns A (2002) Sedation, the doctrine of double effect and the end of life. *Int J Palliat Nurs* **8**(7): 341–3

Twycross R, Wilcock A, Charlesworth S, Dickman A (2002) *Palliative Care Formularly.* 2nd edn. Radcliffe Medical Press, Oxford

Wilkinson J (1995) Ethical issues in palliative care. In: Doyle D, Hanks GWC, Macdonald N (eds) *Oxford Textbook of Palliative Medicine.* Oxford University Press, Oxford

CHAPTER 13

Multi-faith chaplaincy

Andy SJ Lie

Britain is both a community of citizens and a community of communities, both a liberal and a multicultural society, and needs to reconcile their sometimes conflicting requirements.
The Future of Multi-Ethnic Britain (The Parekh Report, 2000: ix)

If one undertakes a brief survey of recent advertisements of NHS hospital chaplaincy posts, an anomaly immediately becomes clear: these advertisements, which mostly, if not all, appear in publications such as the national weekly *Church Times*, seek applications from ordained ministers from the main Christian denominations in Britain. This means that if you are a priest or an ordained minister with a requisite minimum number of years of 'pastoral experience' from the Anglican, Roman-Catholic or Free Churches (which includes the Methodist, Baptist and the United Reformed churches), then you will be eligible to apply.

This dominant and essentially unjust paradigm of recruitment needs to be reviewed and challenged on many fronts:

- Most of these chaplaincy departments in NHS Trusts purport to be 'multi-faith', yet it is clear that for the main chaplain and chaplaincy manager posts, only Christian ministers are eligible to apply. A further cause for injustice is the fact that, with the Church of England as the established church, the majority of chaplaincy manager or team-leader posts remain in the hands of Anglican priests.
- As far as the process of chaplaincy appointments is concerned, we need to ask why secular establishments such as NHS Trusts need to be 'controlled' continually by the Christian church, not least in post-Christian and multi faith Britain. The church, through the Hospital Chaplaincies Council, will argue that this is primarily to ensure the maintaining of professional standards, as is the case with other healthcare professionals, such as nurses. However, it is both probable and reasonable that professional

standards could be maintained without the purview of ecclesiastical authorities, even though chaplains themselves are strictly not healthcare professionals.

■ There is hardly any scope for lay persons (that is, those who are not ordained in any church) to apply, reinforcing the traditional but mistaken belief that religious, spiritual and pastoral care is the sole domain of ordained ministers. This often detracts from the fact that many lay persons do have valuable pastoral and other experiences to offer to hospital chaplaincy.

■ It is clear that potential applicants from the other major world faiths are excluded from applying. This is argued on the basis that the predominant patient population is assumed to be Christian. Hence, there is hardly any justification to appoint people from other world faiths to full-time posts unless they can show that there are numerically 'sufficient' patients from these world faiths in the hospitals. Another corollary is that managerial posts are even further from the grasp of potential chaplains from other world faiths.

■ Last, but not least, the most important factor alluded to earlier that needs considering is: why are advertisements limited to the church press? Chaplaincy advertisements hardly, if ever, appear in the *Health Service Journal*, the mainstream broadsheet newspapers or the various established community publications. This practice ensures that chaplaincy posts are primarily limited to Christian ministers and therefore there is a false perception that there is no need to advertise elsewhere. Furthermore, the persons involved in the actual recruitment process are limited to departmental managers, personnel officers and ministers from a Christian tradition rather than from diverse backgrounds.

Although the demands on hospital chaplaincy are ever increasing, chaplaincy services themselves remain very traditional and Christian in the main. In the rest of this chapter, I shall discuss a number of key issues related to the notion of 'multi-faith chaplaincy' and how the NHS itself could propel this particular service into the twenty-first century.

Multi-faith chaplaincy — is it really possible?

It is important at the outset to address the question of whether the notion of 'multi-faith chaplaincy' itself is possible, let alone feasible. We also need to ask if traditional Christian chaplaincies are actually willing to change so as to pave the way for genuine multi-faith approaches and workings.

I am sure that, while many in the NHS wish to see a real change, the fact remains that for the foreseeable future, religious and spiritual care will continue under the domain of Christian chaplaincies. In any acute NHS Trust, the bulk of chaplaincy sessions remain Christian, usually shared among the major denominations. In this context, we need to note that there has been a substantial increase in ecumenical cooperation over the years, resulting in a decreased Anglican dominance. On the other hand, very few paid sessions, if any, are allocated to the other world faiths.

From my experience of working in three acute trusts in Birmingham, UK, the reality is that, to speak metaphorically, the size of the cake remains the same, but a radical carving out is needed so that other world faiths could get a decent slice. There would therefore appear to be an urgent need for more resources to be committed to employing chaplains from other world faiths. But these resources are difficult to come by in the cash-strapped NHS, where managers are constantly pressed to produce results alongside the incessant drive for meeting targets.

An innovative suggestion was put to me by a Birmingham community leader. It may be possible to appoint a full-time chaplain of a world faith (for example, a Sikh) who could work across a few hospitals, each with a small percentage of staff and patients from that faith. Although there will be logistical difficulties to overcome, together with the coordinating of the financial machinery, this approach could potentially bring together the various chaplaincies and hospitals in a creative partnership. However, we are far from such innovations. Instead, what we are seeing is what we have been relying on for a very long time in the NHS — that is, that chaplaincies generally capitalising on a vital resource for Christian needs.

Without volunteers, such as the Women's Royal Voluntary Service (WRVS), the NHS in general could grind to a halt. The Christian volunteers have themselves traditionally played a key role within the chaplaincy service. We are now beginning to see some encouraging signs as individuals from other world faiths serve as chaplaincy volunteers. However, the services of these volunteers should not be solely relied upon to meet the needs of patients from minority-faith communities. In the long term, this should never be an alternative to officially paid staff. The danger of this practice is that it can exploit other world-faiths volunteers who provide a service that is free, and indefinite. An underlying assumption therefore needs to be challenged here — that because the model of Christian volunteers has worked well for so long, this can be extrapolated to other world-faiths volunteers who will willingly work to this model.

It is disingenuous, though certainly not uncommon, to note the claim (especially in chaplaincy-post advertisements such as those mentioned in the introduction) that a certain department is 'multi-faith'. However, it is far from clear how many purportedly 'multi-faith' chaplaincies actually have paid staff from other world faiths. Many have at best one or two part-time staff from other religious communities (often Muslim), while the rest are predominantly Christian. My experience is that many chaplaincies merely hold a list of contacts of local faith communities and their religious leaders whom they can call on for help regularly and frequently in emergencies.

The implications are clear. On the one hand, part-time Muslim chaplains (for example) will remain part-time and resources are never available to increase their hours. (I say this with some frustration because a Muslim chaplain I helped to appoint has remained in the same part-time arrangement for the past four years and it has seemed almost 'impossible' to give him a half-time appointment, despite a visible increase in workload from this faith.) On the other hand, it is very difficult for the part-time chaplains' views to be heard at higher levels of the organisation, let alone for them to have any sort of coordinating or managing role. Responsibility for major decisions will continue to rest with the Christian chaplaincy manager or team leader, who is most likely to be Anglican.

An issue that can raise much discussion in any multi-faith chaplaincy is that of terminology. Up to now, I have used the terms 'chaplain' and 'chaplaincy' quite loosely. These terms have a Christian origin and a wide usage. Over the years, they have been increasingly borrowed by other world faiths (for example, in British prison settings). I often wonder if there are more neutral terms such as 'spiritual care givers' or 'religious advisers', which could be meaningfully used. Obviously, this begs an important question about who in the modern hospital setting is the locus of spiritual care. Would it be the nurse, doctor, other healthcare professional or the chaplain? Spiritual care should be an integral part of holistic care and therefore all care-givers have spiritual responsibilities.

If, for the sake of discussion, a different term like 'imam' is used, what status will that Muslim person have alongside the Christian chaplain in the ward? The fact is, as things are at present, most if not all patients and staff are so used to the term 'chaplain' that other terms will catch on in common parlance only with great difficulty. A practical way out of this is to use both terms. For example, a Muslim religious functionary, with the requisite training, could use the term 'imam' as a title before his name, and beneath that he could professionally adopt the term 'Muslim Chaplain'.

Conversely, if the universal term 'chaplain' is used for everyone, does it in any way compromise the distinctiveness of each of the other world faiths? I personally do not think so. However, what is potentially compromising or even damaging is that, if different terms are used for different faiths, only those with the title of a 'chaplain' (especially in the case of Christian priests or ordained ministers) will be acknowledged, while others may be relegated to a second- or third-class existence. Furthermore, as far as patients and staff are concerned, remembering that the former are most vulnerable in any hospital or hospice setting, a diversity of terms will only give rise to unnecessary confusion.

Be that as it may, the key issue remains that of access for patients and staff within the NHS to the proper provision of multi-faith religious and spiritual care. This dire shortfall has been attested by a 2003 survey (Gatrad, Sadiq and Sheikh). It is crucial at this juncture to consider briefly what official sanctions are given to improve the situation within NHS hospitals.

Setting in the wider context — official guidelines

It is a well-worn truism enshrined in *The Patient's Charter* (1991) that the standard of service that a patient can expect to receive in both primary and secondary care is that his or her privacy, dignity, religious and cultural beliefs are to be respected at all times and in all places. This rhetoric is laudable, but we all know that the reality is otherwise. Then, in 1992, the Health Service guidelines, *Meeting the Spiritual Needs of Patients and Staff* (DoH, 1992), were issued by the Management Executive, making some useful recommendations for the provision of religious and spiritual care. In both letter and spirit, these guidelines were clearly intent on 'multi-faith' approaches and did not favour Christianity. However, it has long been recognised that this guidance has still not ensured a proper multi-faith provision of religious and spiritual care.

After many years of consultation, the Department of Health (DoH) finally issued the key document *NHS Chaplaincy: Meeting the Religious and Spiritual Needs of Patients and Staff: Guidance for Managers and those Involved in the Provision of Chaplaincy-Spiritual Care* (2003). This has certainly been an improvement on the 1992 guidelines. It is a culmination of many years of discussion and consultation via the Multi-Faith Group for Healthcare Chaplaincy, whose chair was from the Baha'i faith. It is purportedly a 'best practice guide' covering a whole range of key issues, including a framework for chaplaincy-spiritual care; chaplaincy appointments; data protection; volunteers; sacred spaces; training and development; bereavement services; and emergency planning.

Unfortunately, it is on the whole an anodyne document and I cannot hide my disappointment with it. Although interspersed with some concrete examples taken from NHS Trusts, the various sections are really quite thin with recommendations and guidelines stating the obvious. Moreover, the rather general section on 'framework for calculation of total chaplaincy-spiritual care time' (a three-stage process) really does not go far enough to ensure adequate multi-faith provision. I cannot help but feel that this document, though eagerly awaited, is not sufficiently robust and would perpetuate the lip-service currently paid to multi-faith approaches in chaplaincy services.

Perhaps the one useful thing from the document is already hinted in the title. For the future, the service is no longer to be called 'chaplaincy' but 'chaplaincy-spiritual care'. Admittedly, it will be interesting to see the workings of this document within the NHS alongside a much more substantial document, also released in November 2003, on chaplaincy and spiritual-healthcare workforce development (SYWDC, 2003).

Where do we go from here?

I believe that a major assumption from the previous discussion is the nature of spiritual and religious needs in a modern post-Christian society like Britain. In particular, in British multi-faith society, it is vital that different models of spiritual and religious care are sought. We need to move away from the traditional focus of a Christian priest offering 'pastoral care', where the term itself implies a strong Judaeo-Christian bias.

This raises two questions. First, how do we resist the pressure to mold other world faiths according to the Christian approach? Second, are circumstances sufficiently conducive for new models of spiritual care to evolve naturally?

If this is the framework that we are working within, who and what should hospital senior managers look for when they recruit and retain members of other world faiths to complement the work of Christian chaplains? Is it always necessary to have a theologically or religiously qualified person? I believe that we should creatively seek other possibilities — the social worker, link worker, counsellor, teacher, community specialist, healthcare professional — each with a deeply held religious faith and practice. This raises two further questions. First, how do we assess the suitability of these potential candidates when they do come forward? Second, will they be able to obtain organisational support for the spiritual and religious care they will undertake?

These are important practical issues for consideration for any NHS Trust that is serious about considering a multi-faith spiritual-care approach. With reference to the questions above, I am not referring simply to the staff support within the hospital, but, crucially, support available within the communities. In many major British cities, there is now in existence some form of a partnership among the various religious communities. Hence, if a Council of Faiths is set up, this could serve as a first point of contact for the NHS Trust concerned. Furthermore, approaching the issue in this manner may add strength to the idea that the public sector is willing to collaborate with communities (be they faith-based or minority-ethnic), which so often could be patronised when it comes to consultation and the delivery of services.

A related but no less important issue is that of worship and sacred spaces. We need to ask what an NHS Trust's responsibility is for this provision alongside any involvement from the religious communities. The further development of sacred spaces in the current NHS hospital settings is fraught with thorny issues. Although Christian spaces, be they in the form of a Victorian chapel guarded by inflexible rules or a modern user-friendly adaptable room, have been made available for use in most hospitals, the provision of specific religious spaces for the major world religions has always met with obstacles and opposition.

It is only in recent years that NHS management has begun to see the need for the provision of spaces for both patients and staff from the other world faiths. However, space is still at a premium. What is most likely to happen in many hospitals, for example, is the setting-up of a 'multi-faith room', usually next to the chapel. In practice, this 'multi-faith room' is normally set aside for people of all faiths besides Christianity. This approach is quite insidious, although good intentions abound. Whereas in the earlier discussion on chaplaincy services, 'multi-faith' predominantly meant a Christian department with some very loosely attached persons from other world faiths, 'multi-faith' in current sacred-space discussion and practice could mean 'anything other than Christian'. This blatant shift in understanding of 'multi-faith' is remarkable.

Some principal concerns

In the light of the above discussion, one can easily become pessimistic. But there are six important developments worth highlighting, even if their discussion is rather limited in this short chapter.

First of all, it is crucial to recognise that there is no level playing field (Lie, 2001). At the end of the day, even in post-Christian Britain, chaplaincy services in the NHS will be predominantly staffed and serviced by Christians. It is extremely difficult to alter this state of affairs, especially in view of the continuing establishment of the Church of England and despite the improvement in ecumenical relations over the years.

This leads to the second brief point about power relations between the church and other world faiths. It is inevitable that there will never be a balance of power so long as the Church, which often claims to speak for the majority, 'calls the shots' in matters spiritual, even if they are within a secular institution like the NHS. As hinted in the previous section, the lack of a balance of power will also lead to exploitation, not least in terms of influencing how other world faiths should adapt their *modus operandi* according to the 'majority'. There is another insidious twist to this particular point in terms of practicality (or, many would indeed argue, the time-honoured integrity of Christian chaplaincy), whereby Christian chaplains are prone to providing 'generic chaplaincy', while other world-faiths chaplains are confined to their respective patients and staff. Here, we should be alert to the ethical considerations where a confusion of professional roles on the part of Christian chaplains could lead to highly inadequate religious and spiritual care (Engelhardt Jr, 1998).

Third, although the Human Rights Act (1998) and the Race Relations (Amendment) Act (2001), together with other EU Employment Equality directives (2003–2006) are fully operational, there is still the risk that the legislation will be open to infringement. For example, assuming an NHS Trust is willing to provide even the very basic services for a faith group, be they patients or staff, that intention must be matched by proper outcomes. If the services do not adequately produce an acceptable outcome, then the adverse impact will be felt by that group. Hence, providing a Muslim prayer room is well-intentioned but if it only has space for four persons at any one time and without proper ablutions facilities, it will adversely affect Muslim staff and patients if this group constitutes a fairly large percentage of people in the hospital. Hence, good intentions and token measures will not do. I foresee that new landmark cases will be tested in the courts in years to come when the new Commission for Equality and Human Rights is finally established.

Fourth, in post-Christian Britain, there needs to be much more research into and writing on religious and spiritual care in medical and health contexts from multi-faith perspectives. Hitherto, the field has seen an abundance of works emanating from a Christian perspective or with a Christian bias. In reality, 'the health care understanding of "spirituality" is a secularized version of the Christian understanding of spirituality' (Markham, 1998: 74). In practice, however, this can often end up in a kind of nebulous 'healthcare spirituality' without the necessary religious underpinnings. In other words, 'healthcare spirituality' could quite easily fall into the pragmatic trap of thinking, 'if it works for me, then it's absolutely fine'. As was alluded to in a previous section, I am not saying that there is no place for such an approach to spirituality, but what is needed is care in situating 'spirituality' alongside real religious and spiritual needs, lest its lack of religious underpinnings be an affront to others from deeply held religious traditions. We also need to engage at the same time with the various humanist and pagan traditions that are now gaining recognition and capacity in Britain.

Fifth, alongside solid research and writing, is the need for good and proper data collection of patients' and staff members' religious or non-religious affiliations (for example, as has happened at the Acorns Children's Hospices, Birmingham: see *Chapter 10*). Obviously, these need to be collected within the bounds of patient consent and confidentiality, and under Caldicott Guardianship. All this should not detract from the fact that good, diverse and inclusive data are crucial for solid research to be done. Furthermore, we need to go beyond data collection — future research must include in-depth qualitative approaches where views and experiences concerned with religious and spiritual matters are as accurately collected as possible. This will necessarily feed into a narrative approach in health and medicine which is currently being promoted as part of holistic care. In this regard, a significant collection like Greenhalgh and Hurwitz (1998) provides the much-needed insights into this narrative approach, which in turn facilitates stories of illness and dying alongside developing our understanding of spirituality. Sensitivity to multicultural nuances within specialist palliative care and hospice services has been effective in eliciting fresh perspectives on 'truth', death, patient autonomy and professional control (McNamara, 2001).

Last but not least, in relation to the undue enshrinement of 11th September 2001 ('9/11') and the subsequent atrocities in Bali, Madrid and London ('7/7') into our historical consciousness, I believe it is now crucial to address head-on matters of discrimination and Islamophobia. For good or for bad, we are still feeling the impact of the tragedies in these cities, but this must be seen in the wider context of injustice and 'neo-imperialism'. Nevertheless, Muslims in general have felt very vulnerable, especially as a result of the so-called 'anti-terror' legislation promulgated in Britain in the past three years. We need to be aware of our own inner views, racism and prejudices. It is therefore timely to remind ourselves that, in this discussion of multi-faith chaplaincy, critical training with regard to the understanding and appreciation of 'the Other' is ever more pressing. In particular, with reference to Islam and Muslims, and against the prevailing climate of prejudice and hatred, there needs to be genuine recognition that understanding and practice of wholeness, care, spirituality and ethics have their roots in a rich civilisation (Rahman, 1993; Visscher, 2005). Not to recognise the historical and geographical far-reaching effects of Islamic medical and healthcare traditions and practices is to fly in the face of human decency and dignity.

Conclusion

I hope I have sufficiently shown that the prospect for minority-faiths chaplains is not bright, as things stand in the NHS. The rhetoric of official guidance is one thing — but the reality is proving otherwise in the current business-driven climate of the NHS. Nevertheless, there is an urgent need for the voices of these minority-faiths chaplains to be heard so that they may creatively contribute to the development of proper multi-faith chaplaincies in the future.

Three main areas need addressing. The first is the willingness of Christian chaplaincy managers to involve minority-faiths chaplains in major decision-making, business-planning, policy-development and managerial responsibility. The second area is to involve them directly in the planning and delivery of training sessions so that healthcare staff especially are both introduced and acquainted with new and fresh perspectives. The third is the outreach potential held by the minority-faiths chaplains to the surrounding communities, in the hope that good relations are built between those who provide healthcare services and those who receive them. Needless to say, the voices of minority-faiths patients and staff need airing too. Without these voices 'from the margins', any future development and progress will only prove that the dominant paradigm — that is, Christian-based and, in some cases, even racist — will prevail.

Bearing in mind that there are many other philosophical issues to consider, I have consciously attempted a practical approach to this discussion of the relevant issues for multi-faith chaplaincy. At first sight, it may seem to have little bearing on the other chapters in this book. But I hope that when read in the context of other chapters on palliative care, it will eventually provide a useful focal point whereby fresh thinking and discussions could take place concerning the nature of religious and spiritual care in contemporary healthcare contexts.

Key points of *Chapter 13*

- There is clear evidence that the recruitment process for hospital chaplains needs to reflect the true diversity within multi-faith Britain and not pander to Christian hegemonic concerns.
- We must go beyond the misleading rhetoric of 'multi-faith chaplaincy' to see the reality in each NHS Trust/hospital or independent hospice. The current dire state of affairs can only be reversed when secure mainstream resources are committed to recruit more chaplains from the world faiths (other than Christian). This is also to ensure that we pay more than lip-service to improving access to religious and spiritual care for patients and staff.
- Crucial DoH guidelines and policies issued in 1992 and 2003 seem only to perpetuate the status quo rather than provide the radical alternatives that are necessary for the proper implementation of multi-faith chaplaincy services.
- Alongside the provision of resources for a multi-faith chaplaincy, there needs to be a concerted effort to explore new models of religious, pastoral and spiritual care that could potentially evolve from engaging with the world faiths.
- Qualitative approaches in research need to be harnessed and nurtured to allow the stories of illness and dying to surface alongside our developing understandings of spirituality.
- The ground has to be cleared for a much more level playing field in terms of resource-input, recruitment, deployment, progression and broader engagement of chaplains from all the world faiths.

References

Department of Health (DoH) (2003) *NHS Chaplaincy: Meeting the Religious and Spiritual Needs of Patients and Staff: Guidance for Managers and those Involved in the Provision of Chaplaincy-Spiritual Care*. DoH, London

Engelhardt Jr HT (issue ed) (1998) Generic chaplaincy: providing spiritual care in a post-Christian age. *Christ Bioeth* **4**: 231–315

European Union Employment Equality Directives (2003/6) Migration Policy Group, Brussels

Gatrad AR, Sadiq R, Sheikh A (2003) Multifaith chaplaincy. *Lancet* **362**: 748

Gatrad AR, Brown E, Sheikh A (2004) Developing multi-faith chaplaincy. *Arch Dis Child* **89**: 504–05

Greenhalgh T, Hurwitz B (eds) (1998) *Narrative-Based Medicine: Dialogue and Discourse in Clinical Practice.* BMJ Books, London

Lie ASJ (2001) No level playing field: the multi-faith context and its challenges. In: Helen Orchard (ed) *Spirituality in Health Care Contexts.* Jessica Kingsley Publishers, London and Philadephia

McNamara B (2001) *Fragile Lives: Death, Dying and Care.* Open University Press, Buckingham and Philadelphia

Markham I (1998) Spirituality and the world faiths. In: Cobb M, Robshaw V (eds) *The Spiritual Challenge of Health Care.* Churchill Livingstone, Edinburgh

NHS Management Executive (1992) *Meeting the Spiritual Needs of Patients and Staff: Good Practice Guidance.* DoH, London

Parekh B (chair) (2000) *The Future of Multi-Ethnic Britain* (The Parekh Report). Profile Books, London

Rahman F (1993) *Health and Medicine in the Islamic Tradition: Change and Identity.* S Abdul Majeed & Co, Kuala Lumpur

Sheikh A, Gatrad AR, Sheikh U, Panesar SS, Shuja S (2004) Hospital chaplaincy units show bias towards Christianity (letter to editor) *BMJ* **329**: 626

Sheikh A, Panesar SS (2004) Myth of NHS multifaith chaplaincy. *Muslim News* **24 Sept 2004**: 5

South Yorkshire Workforce Development Confederation (SYWDC) (2003) *Caring for the Spirit: a Strategy for the Chaplaincy and Spiritual Healthcare Workforce.* SYWDC, Sheffield, UK

Visscher C (2005) Health care and spirituality: spiritually sensitive care of the terminally ill Muslim patient. *Interreligious Insight: a Journal of Dialogue and Engagement* **3**: 68–77

CHAPTER 14

South-Asian perspectives on bereavement

Shirley Firth

Enable me to be helpful to those in difficulty; kind to those in need; sympathetic to those whose hearts are sore and sad.
   Anon

Palliative care aims to provide holistic care to patients and to support families before and after death, but South-Asian patients have often been neglected, with low rates of referrals and often inadequate provision for specific religious and cultural needs. The roles and needs of family members before and after death are often misunderstood by professionals. Relatives may not be able to facilitate appropriate religious rituals or be able to deal with bureaucratic, legal and financial arrangements, in addition to the organisation of burial or cremation. Separation from their homeland, poverty, fragmentation of the extended family and poor English make bereavement more difficult for South-Asian families who may not therefore receive support during a relative's illness or after their death.

   Professionals often know little about different communities — or even realise just how diverse they are, resulting in bewilderment at unfamiliar attitudes and behaviour. There is little research or written material on cultural aspects of bereavement for minority ethnic people in the diaspora. Apart from anthropological studies, most writings on cross-cultural perspectives on death focus on idealised general information about religious beliefs and practices (see Irish *et al*, 1993; Parkes *et al*, 1997; Morgan and Laungani, 2002). They thus ignore their complexity, their sociological and psychological dimensions, and the impact of change on the way people grieve and mourn. Writings on trans-cultural psychology and counselling do not deal with bereavement, but provide useful insights into communication and different ways of expressing feelings.

   This chapter examines cultural perspectives on loss and bereavement, drawing on the author's own research into a British Hindu community and subsequently with other South-Asian communities, and suggests ways in which professionals can better understand and help the bereaved.

Identity

A nurse who told me 'I've never nursed any ethnics' was astonished to be told that we are all 'ethnic'. 'Ethnicity' and 'culture' are often used interchangeably, but ethnicity includes shared ancestry, as well as culture and language. Culture reflects the way people view and experience the world and how they behave (Helman, 1994). It is also dynamic and changes in different contexts and times as people adapt to a new environment. Many second-generation immigrants become bi-cultural, straddling both the 'home' and British cultures, but where a group retains its identity, it can be threatening to the majority community.

A vital aspect of culture is religion, which provides a world-view about God or the 'ultimate reality' and the meaning of existence. Both belief systems and practices provide strategies for dealing with death and mourning. People who have moved away from their religion often rediscover meaning in it at times of crisis. The current separation between religion and spirituality may be meaningless to people of faith (Gilliat-Ray, 2003).

We derive our sense of identity from family structures, gender, socio-economic status and education. The death of a family member threatens this identity, exacerbated for many South-Asian immigrants by multiple losses, including loss of home, country, relatives and, for refugees especially, earlier traumatic experiences. According to Eisenbruch, uprooting 'disrupts the continuity of an individual's concept of selfhood... In particular it disrupts the "structures of meaning", defined by Marris as "the conceptual organisation of understanding one's surroundings"' (Eisenbruch II, 1984: 298).

Death of a parent or spouse may represent the loss of a way of life. Parkes' (1986) theory of psycho-social transitions shows how the familiar or 'assumptive' ways of looking at the world are forcibly changed. Separation from the homeland and family may be more acute for older people, especially if the body of the deceased is returned, with no possibility of visiting the grave as occurs in Muslim Pakistani and Bangladeshi communities (Gardner, 1998, 2001; Henley and Schott, 1999).

Expectations of appropriate rituals may be shattered. For example, Muslims may be disturbed by the necessity for a post-mortem and delays in burial. Hindus and Sikhs, who cremate immediately in India, often have to wait a week or more for the funeral in the UK, meaning that the structured mourning period has to happen before the disposal of the body, instead of afterwards.

Family structures

Traditional South-Asian families are 'collectivist', meaning the individual is seen in terms of a 'relational' or 'familial' self (Fielding *et al*, 1998), which affects choices and decision-making. It also has a major impact on grief, which is seen less as a private affair than embedded in a social context. Because of the process of acculturation (the process by which the immigrant culture adapts to the indigenous culture) families cannot always function in the traditional way; nor can it be assumed that they can provide adequate support.

Silverman (2004: 25) discusses the changing status of women when they are widowed: 'If the role of wife is central to a woman's life, what happens when her spouse dies and the role of wife no longer defines her?' In traditional Indian families, a wife lives with her husband's parents following an arranged marriage. Her primary role is to bear sons to continue the lineage, which can lead to an intense bond between mother and son, as his birth validates her identity as a mother (Kakar, 1978). The death of an only son has long-term economic, religious and social implications; he is the 'old-age pension' and guarantor of care throughout old age and, for Hindus, of a secure place in the next life through rites after death. The premature death of the husband may be blamed on the wife, and without adult sons, she can be isolated, shunned and considered permanently unlucky and impure.

The loss of a parent may also be profoundly disorientating because of the authority structure within the family. According to Kakar (1978: 36), 'Autonomy arouses the most severe of the culturally supported anxieties — the fear of isolation and estrangement that are visited upon the completely autonomous human being'. After death, the son or daughter may 'assume a set of social obligations as prescribed by his/her ethnic group' (Eisenbruch, 1988: II: 325), identifying more strongly with the beliefs of the parent and culture.

Grief and mourning

'Grief' is an emotion that arises in response to loss of a significant person, often with psychological and physical manifestations: '"Mourning" is the way in which this is manifested, often in culturally determined ways, and usually for a specified time in a particular society, with cultural variations in how far particular kinds of grief experiences are legitimated or frowned on, and which types of relationships justify its expression or demand its suppression' (Parkes and Weiss, 1983: 2). Bereavement is 'both the period of time following a death, during which grief occurs, and also the state of experiencing grief' (Rosenblatt *et al*, 1976: 2).

There has been considerable debate as to whether people from different cultures feel, express and experience grief differently. It is difficult to extrapolate theories from one culture and apply them to another. Because of wide variations in the way people behave, some sociologists and anthropologists argue that grief is socially constructed, implying that society determines not just how we should behave, but what we actually feel (Radcliffe Brown, 1964; Durkheim, 1965; Seale, 1998).

Stroebe and Schut suggest, however, that there is empirical evidence from biological studies that there are similar emotions of grief in all human beings, which 'provide the fundamental background from which cultural variations should be viewed' (Stroebe and Schut, 1998: 7). In the past, psychological approaches have focused more on individuals and have been influenced by Freud, Lindemann (1944) and others who view grief as a disorder from which the person must become detached from the lost one to recover.

The theories of Stages (Kubler-Ross, 1969) and Tasks (Worden, 1991) have been useful tools for understanding how the bereaved 'work' through their loss, by accepting it, experiencing the pain and adjusting to a newly ordered environment. However, these concepts are often used prescriptively with an assumption that the person must 'move on'. Such approaches have been criticised as 'ethnocentric', particularly as they focus on the individual mourner. Western ideas about 'normal' or 'pathological' grief may be totally inappropriate for South Asians, as in some circumstances repression of emotions and memories may be adaptive. Stroebe's and Schut's (1998) dual-process model of grieving, on the other hand, allows for cultural variations in which at times there is an orientation towards loss, 'letting go of the past', and at other times an orientation towards restoration, remaining with or keeping hold of the deceased.

Both the dual-process model and the interactionist approach may be more appropriate in a cross-cultural context, where the community takes priority over the individual. The latter recognises the influence of social contexts and places 'particular emphasis on communication and meaning of how these affect the experiences of (dying) patients, their relatives and others close to them, and those caring for them' (Field, Hockey and Small, 1997: 23). Silverman (2004: 26) and also sees grief as an 'interactive process involving multiple mourners and others in the lives of these mourners, highlighting how mutuality and interdependence are expressed in their world-view as well as in their daily lives'. This also allows for locating the dead in a societal context — not only allowing discussions about the deceased (Walter, 1999), but also placing them in heaven or creating an ancestor, and maintaining continuing bonds thereafter: an important aspect of life for many cultures, for example, Hindus. This also acknowledges the validity of people's experiences of the presence of the dead, without reducing them to 'hallucinations' (see Parkes, 1986).

Western ways of categorising and understanding emotional and somatic conditions need to be treated with caution. For example, 'guilt' may have different connotations for a Christian and a Hindu, particularly in the light of concepts such as Karma (deeds) and Kismat (fate). It is worth pointing out here that Chinese and Japanese cultures focus more on shame than on guilt. When researching British Hindu approaches to death (Firth, 1997), I found many similar classic Western patterns of grief describing numbness, denial, anger and so on, but with a significant difference: religious teachings in all the Asian traditions discourage violent emotions; but, in reality, I found that there are outbursts of violent emotion from the outset, often with social expectations to weep publicly during condolence visits and at funerals.

Emotional reactions

The expression of feelings may seem extreme in some cultures, but in others repression is quite normal. Bali and Egypt both have Islamic cultures; in Egypt, grief is expressed overtly and often, in the case of a son's death, for years. The women display 'intense, heart-rending grieving... Females will scream, yell, beat their breasts, collapse in each others' arms and be quite beyond themselves for days, even weeks on end' (Wikan, 1988: 452).

In Bali, grief has to be controlled and contained because it is 'contagious and detrimental to all', including the soul of the deceased (Wikan, 1988: 456). For Hindus, excessive emotion may result in the deceased's ghost hanging around and harming the living or failing to reach its goal. For example, a dying Punjabi woman said, 'Don't cry, your tears will make a river for me to cross' (see *Chapter 5, Panel 5.1*).

Wikan suggests that it is culture and other variables rather than religion that determine behaviour, but this is also influenced by other factors such as social rank, age and gender. While Queen Victoria's endless mourning is sometimes described as pathological, for many Hindu widows, as for Egyptian mothers, and for many from other cultures, devotion to the deceased is expected to be life long and is 'normal'.

Depression may not be recognised or acknowledged by South Asians. Life gives Sukh (happiness) and Dukh (sadness) and what matters is how a person copes with both on the path to salvation (Krause, 1989). There are deep-seated taboos against expressing anger against a dead husband, older brother or parent, and in my research, no-one reported feelings of anger against relatives (other than two aunts who were deemed to have gone straight to hell. One, it was assumed, would be reborn as a vulture!). However, many of my informants felt anger against medical staff for exclusion, racism, failure to provide appropriate care, and lack of open communication.

Many older Hindu and Sikh widows internalise traditional social attitudes by classing themselves as 'unlucky' and 'impure', to the extent that they do not join in any social functions (Firth, 1997, 1999; Kalsi, 1996). Young Bangladeshi and Sikh widows are also vulnerable to criticism and unwanted attention. It cannot be assumed, therefore, that those South Asians who are part of extended families will always 'care and support their own'.

Mourning

All South-Asian traditions have established mourning patterns, which will vary somewhat according to families and sects. For Hindus and Sikhs, this period lasts for ten or more days, while relatives and neighbours bring food. Hindus withdraw for a given period from society, with a series of elaborate rituals to create a new body for the dead, culminating in a remarkable act of reincorporation in which he or she becomes an ancestor. As for the Sikhs, the mourning period concludes with the gift of a turban to the eldest son to signify he is now the head of the family. Muslims have three days of intense mourning followed by a lesser period of forty days. Muslim widows do not mingle socially outside the family during this period (Idat), at the end of which the Qur'an is read and a feast provided.

Such rituals amongst South Asians give meaning to death and help create a stable and safe place for the mourners. These culturally accepted periods legitimise social withdrawal and the expression of grief. They provide a ritual framework of purposeful activity. The whole process of Afsos (giving regrets) gives both the immediately bereaved and their entire kinship network an opportunity to review and comment on the fullness of the deceased person's life through a structural, verbal and conceptual framework within which everyone can express the many dimensions of their grief.

Sorrow at the loss of a beloved person is only one aspect of mourning. Constant reference 'to the inscrutable powers of the Ultimate' gives meaning and significance to the life of the deceased (Ballard: in Firth, 1997: 154). Narratives about this death and that of others have the function of maintaining and passing on the tradition as a source of inspiration and meaning, and as a way of retaining the deceased as a member of the family. Religious readings, homilies and shared stories about other people's bereavements place death in a context of universal experience, reminding the mourners that death is God's will and that the whole process is in His hands.

One Punjabi woman commented that these narratives were really helpful — and that suffering should therefore not be in solitude. She cited a Hindu version of a Buddhist story of Gotami in which a woman asks a holy man to heal her dead child. He tells her to go to every house that has not known death and bring back a cup of water. She returns empty handed. 'See, in every house death has come'.

Finding meaning

The type of death has a major impact on grieving. A 'good death', in which the person dies consciously and willingly, with his or her mind on God and a belief in continuity, gives meaning to dying and helps the bereaved to know that they have fulfilled their sacred obligations. Such an experience lends itself to subsequent narratives. Many Hindus and Sikhs take comfort from the belief that their deceased relative is reborn, sometimes in the same family, or is 'with God'. For Muslims, the final act of Sakrat, whereby there is reaffirmation of faith, has enormous significance to the dying and his or her relatives (see *Chapter 4*).

It is more difficult to find meaning in 'bad deaths', when the relatives are unable to perform the right rituals and prayers, and to say goodbye properly. A Gujarati family, who were forbidden by the doctor to give Ganges water to a dying aunt 'in case she choked', believed that her ghost would haunt the family for seven generations because this purifying last rite had been omitted (see *Chapter 5*). They had not managed to explain that only a tiny drop was needed, and their pleas were ignored, despite their good English.

The final moments of life have a profoundly spiritual as well as emotional aspect for many people. Gardner (2001) cites Muslim Bangladeshi widows who were sent home during the final hours of their husbands' lives, only to miss being at the deathbed. Those who could bring their husbands home — a sacred space — provide the right prayers and readings, and say farewell, had profound psychological advantages for themselves and the whole family. Among my Hindu and Sikh respondents, those who had the most difficult bereavements were those who were not present at the death and were unable to hear the last words of their relative, or to fulfil their sacred obligations. Some also reported a dismal failure by staff to understand their religious and emotional needs. Many professionals, clearly, do not appreciate the bonds (and constraints) of the extended family, or the immense importance of religion to them at times of crisis.

People of faith may still have existential and spiritual questions of meaning, and seek metaphysical answers, which may be harder to explore outside their own cultural setting. It may also be difficult to share with a co-religionist for fear of being thought of as lacking faith (*Panel 14.1*). This Hindu woman struggled to find meaning and understanding in her faith, not blind acquiescence to a set of doctrines. The phrase 'It is God's will' is said to Hindus, Sikhs and Muslims alike to explain suffering, illness and death. Ballard observes that this

---

Panel 14.1: Why?

A Hindu woman, with a deep faith, still asked the perennial question 'why' when her husband died:

Why did God have to take him away when he was so young? Why doesn't God come and help when the person wants to live, when he is doing so many good things in his life? My husband was so religious, he prayed every day, not in temple or shrine, but a few minutes at bed time... God helps people — why didn't he help us? Bad characters do well, why do good people die?

(Firth, 1997: 196)

---

is not an expression of fatalism, but an exploratory remark inviting discussion and dialogue, implying that one will eventually come to see that it is God's will — part of a divine plan, or 'as in the story of Job, part of an educational theodicy' (Dein and Stygall, 1997: 296).

For the Muslim, peace can only be found by submitting to death gracefully. Kemp, researching Kurds and other Muslims in the USA, found that these communities saw individualistic meaning as less important than a life 'in lived faith, the community of the faithful, and family. Hope is available in abundance for believers' (Kemp, 1996: cited in Gilliat-Ray, 2003: 9).

Bereavement support

Many minority ethnic people need bereavement support, which is rarely available (Spruyt, 1999; Netto *et al*, 2001). Even in closely knit communities, there may be issues that cannot be discussed within the family and social group for reasons of confidentiality (Spruyt, 1999; Somerville, 2001). For example, a Sikh woman had two sons with Duchenne muscular dystrophy. When one died, her husband was so devastated that she had to support him emotionally, and did not tell anyone how she felt. Illnesses such as AIDS and some forms of cancer are so stigmatising that the family becomes isolated.

Older women, who have been dependent on their husbands with restricted access to the outside world, may be thrust into a new world which they have to negotiate without experience or language skills. There may be acute issues of isolation and poverty (Burrows, 1997) and help needed with bureaucracy, property, legal matters, social security and social services. Even with adequate provision, there may be ignorance of services, particularly since terms such as 'bereavement counselling' are not readily translatable into other languages. Bereavement services may be seen as for white Britons only. The idea of asking for help and going outside the family may seem foreign, and there may be anxiety in case this brings shame on the person and family requesting it (Burrows, 1997; Shoaib and Peel, 2003). Further concerns may be the risk of discrimination, language difficulties and lack of cultural sensitivity from service providers.

Bereavement training

The purpose of bereavement support is to 'provide a safe place where feelings can be expressed and accepted, and to assure the client that these feelings are normal and that he or she is not going mad' (Walter, 1999: 197). The counsellor or supporter must grasp the complexities of the cultural context of the bereaved, with some knowledge of intercultural counselling theory, practice and communication.

Much UK intercultural counselling theory and training focuses primarily on racial issues with little reference to bereavement, loss, culture or religion (Kareem and Littlewood, 1992). This disadvantages black counsellors, since 'terms such as "intercultural" have often come to be understood in practice, as "How to work with black clients" [which] to a black trainee... might not be considered as intercultural work at all' (Taylor-Mohammed, 2001: 10).

Transcultural work also has to take into account the client's background, gender, role and place in the family (Currer, 2001). Training should include information about diversity, health issues, social contexts, religion, culture and cultural competence, enabling the supporter to lay aside his or her own cultural expectations and be willing to enter that of the client or client groups (see *Chapter 1*). Netto *et al* (2001) found that mainstream agencies expected counsellors to learn about the relevance of cultural and religious issues from their clients, whereas the 'black-led' organisations stressed the importance of understanding the clients' cultural and religious background before they embarked on counselling.

Intercultural training for bereavement support is sparse and inadequate, often just a single session of a few hours. Spiritual needs, and the value of religious practice and beliefs, as coping strategies must be understood (Burrows, 1997). If supporters or counsellors appear to hold different beliefs and values, the client may feel inhibited about openly expressing fears and emotions (Bahl, 1996). Remaining non-judgemental may be difficult for those who have no religious beliefs and cannot empathise with those who hold different world-views. This requires cultural competence, maintaining a balance 'between not overlooking our shared and universal human characteristics and needs, attributing all the client's problems to some "cultural" peculiarity on the one hand, and on the other, neglecting cultural variability with the aim of treating everyone the same' (Arnold, 1992: 158; Leininger, 1996; Shoaib and Peel, 2003). Western expectations of autonomy and independence may not conform to clients'

Panel 14.2: Unexpected insights from a counselling session

The client attending for bereavement counselling may reveal other issues that are causing distress:

A young Asian woman was referred to me following her mother's death. She did not wish to go to an Asian counsellor for reasons of confidentiality, and she was afraid of being told what she ought to do in line with community attitudes. She had a good degree, and an excellent job, which she abandoned to look after her dying mother and five siblings. What emerged was not just her grief for her mother — a deeply loving woman, who had held the family together — but also her conflict with her father, her own inner self being torn between her love of and sense of duty to her siblings, reinforced strongly by the local community, and her longing for an independent life. She realised that she might never be able to marry her Asian fiancé. Her dominating and abusive father insisted she remain at home to care for her siblings, and she did not dare leave them on their own with him, as they were afraid of him.

(Firth, 2004: 193)

---

expectations of gender roles, and should not affect judgement of women clients (*Panel 14.2*). This young Asian woman's cultural and religious background offered her a strong sense of duty and commitment, but her Western education showed her a wider range of options, so that she was torn between her own independence, her fear of her father, community pressures and her love of her siblings. She did not want 'advice', but an opportunity to explore the issues confronting her.

White workers may be anxious about 'not being accepted by the client', of 'being called racist' and of 'not being able to understand' or 'not being understood', or seen as prying when knowledge of the family's relationships is essential. This needs careful supervision if it is not to paralyse the visitor (Arnold, 1992: 156). Gunaratnam *et al* (1998) suggest these interactions have to involve 'emotional labour', taking informed risks and trusting intuition. It is important to be honest about one's own stereotyping and unconscious racist attitudes. Relevant self-questioning about the latter might be 'Am I being racist?' or 'Am I making inappropriate cultural assumptions about needs and experiences?' Self-monitoring, as well as welcoming feedback from colleagues, carers and patients is recommended. In addition, 'referential grounding' enables one to see the other person as a similar human being, through empathetic awareness, which 'helps to identify ethnic-minority people not as Others, but with common needs and experiences' (Gunaratnam *et al*, 1998: 124).

Occasionally, there is no apparent common experience. People with no religious beliefs may find it difficult to empathise with clients who have radically different world-views about religion and the 'unseen' world. 'The new, rather secularised, individualistic, humanistic definitions of spirituality can mean anything to anyone, regardless of their belief or lack of it, and it is questionable that this makes them useful to anyone' (Gilliat-Ray, 2003: 7). For example, Muslims are the second biggest community in the world and in the UK, yet their needs for spiritual care are being ignored: '"spirituality" means something to Christians, or the general population at large, whatever their belief or lack of it, while 'religion' of a committed and orthodox kind defines the so-called "spiritual needs" of religious minority groups' (Gilliat-Ray, 2003: 10).

In addition, cultural myths about Islam, or about asylum seekers, may engender suspicion and prejudice. It is therefore necessary for professionals to go beyond external differences and relate to each other as human beings by learning from inside — to know from real encounters, and not just 'know about'. We also need to know the people we work with outside the healthcare and social systems as we usually live in social isolation from minority ethnic groups, with little experience of them, except in stress situations (Arnold, 1992).

Practical issues

Clients may not be familiar with the concept of 'counselling' from Euro-American perspectives, which may prevent access to bereavement services, although once services are made available and publicised, they are often used (Netto *et al*, 2001). Ideally, counsellors should speak the same language, but some clients may have reservations about confidentiality and fear that people from the same community might know the family. Of equal importance is whether the counsellor or befriender is culturally aware. There may be preference for a South-Asian counsellor from a different community or religion. Ideally, members of the respective communities should undergo training for bereavement support. However, the concept of voluntary service to people outside their own group may not be familiar and may have to be carefully explained.

Netto *et al* (2001: 4) also found that South-Asian clients initially expected advice, but 'when familiar with the nature of the service, the qualities they value most are being "heard" and treated with respect'. They found that black-led agencies were prepared to be more flexible and offer some advice initially, whilst enabling clients to become more autonomous eventually.

The same investigators found that the time boundary of one-hour consultation 'limited the depth and quality of the experience' for some clients, and that some South-Asian women wanted the option of seeing a counsellor at home, which allowed for a process of social familiarisation. Among my own interviewees, 'serious talk' only began after, for example, a cup of tea and general exchange of information. This is important in establishing trust. Changes to this process take time to explain and put into practice. There should be choices regarding the culture, language and gender of the supporter and place to meet. Continuity of care should be available (Burrows, 1997). The family may be ashamed to ask for practical help, but may need information about available services; bureaucracy around disposal, including how to register death, especially during holidays; and when and where to bury or cremate. There may be issues over post-mortems for Muslims; coroners may be more or less flexible over such requirements. For some immigrant elders, these problems may be exacerbated if they are not eligible for state benefits.

Bereavement services vary across the country, influenced by how they began. Some have grown out of social services; in other areas, there are dedicated posts within nursing, counselling, social work, chaplaincy or volunteer coordinators, which makes assessment of the quality of service provided difficult. The Muslim Bereavement Service in Tower Hamlets, London, UK, was established by the City and East London Bereavement Counselling Service and funded by the UK National Lottery and King's Fund. The training encompassed a wider role of giving advice when required, making appropriate referrals and acting as advocates for clients. The Sandwell and Dudley Cruse Bereavement Centre is training some Asians, with further cross-cultural input from a freelance black-Caribbean trainer.

Link-workers, patient advocates and outreach workers have an important role in providing bereavement support as well as interpreting and providing outreach work. At Compton Hospice in Wolverhampton, UK, the Sikh outreach worker may be called upon to support, for example, Chinese or Caribbean patients and their families who are relieved to find a non-white presence. Acorns Children's Hospices in the West Midlands has not only proved outstanding in attracting children from different minority ethnic groups, but has provided a superb service to families, both before and after death (Notta and Warr, 1998; see *Chapter 10*). A key factor here was the appointment of a single South-Asian outreach worker in the early years, extending to workers from Hindu, Muslim and African-Caribbean communities. In addition to running 'support groups' for mothers, fathers, grandparents, teenagers, siblings and clients with specific life-limiting illnesses such as muscular dystrophy, Acorns provides bereavement support in the home for as long as is necessary.

Conclusions

South-Asian families are currently ill-served with bereavement support, and the challenge of providing suitable, culturally competent services involves a wider education in cross-cultural communication, culture and religion. Training should take into account transcultural studies, from ethnographic and psychological perspectives, and be committed to religious, racial and cultural awareness.

A more uniform, coherent and culturally relevant service is needed throughout the country, reflecting the cultural, religious and ethnic mix of the communities they serve. Recruitment of minority ethnic nurses, social workers, counsellors and bereavement visitors should be a priority. With a range of support services there could be choices in type and continuity of support. Publicity and information in appropriate languages need to be developed consistently throughout the country (Burrows, 1997). Policy decision-makers should be aware of the diversity of the local communities, guarding against stereotyping and recognising clients as unique individuals.

A good programme should not only serve clients, but also support health workers and counsellors, who gain immeasurably in understanding and empathising with all clients. In particular, these support workers need to develop cultural curiosity, a willingness to explore and get to know the client groups in their area, and take delight in both the sameness and the stimulus of understanding differences that transcultural relationships brings for client, supporter and counsellor alike.

Key points of *Chapter 14*

- South Asians do not have adequate access to palliative care or bereavement care.
- More appropriate forms of bereavement support for minority ethnic clients are needed.
- There are many different South-Asian religions and cultures; it is important to treat people as individuals and not impose racial or cultural stereotypes on them.
- There is a wide range of 'normal' emotional responses to grief, including crying and wailing, as well as stoicism. There are no fixed times or ways to 'get over it'.
- It cannot be assumed that Western models of grief are appropriate in a South-Asian setting.
- Mourning rituals give religious meaning to death and provide comfort and social stability, as well as ways of returning to social life.
- Intercultural training needs to include insights from cultural psychology.

References

Arnold E (1992) Intercultural social work. In: Kareem J, Littlewood R (eds) *Intercultural Therapy: Themes, Interpretations and Practice*. Blackwell, Oxford

Bahl Veena (1996a) Cancer and ethnic minorities — the Department of Health's perspective. *Br J Cancer* **74**(Suppl XXIX): S2–S10

Burrows A (1997) Bereavement, culture and counselling: five Asian perspectives on issues affecting bereaved people of Pakistani descent living in Britain today, and implications for a bereavement counselling service. MA dissertation, Manchester University

Currer C (2001) Is grief an illness? Issues of theory in relation to cultural diversity and the grieving process. In: Hockey J, Katz J, Small N (eds) *Grief, Mourning and Death Ritual*. Open University Press, Buckingham

Dein S, Stygall J (1997) Does being religious help or hinder coping with chronic illness? A critical literature review. *Palliat Med* **11**: 291–8

Durkheim E (1919) *The Elementary Forms of the Religious Life*. Unwin, London

Eisenbruch M (1984) Cross-cultural aspects of bereavement II: ethnic and cultural variations in the development of bereavement practices. *Cult Med Psychiatry* **8**(4): 315–47

Field D, Hockey J, Small N (eds) (2001) *Grief, Mourning and Death Ritual*. Open University Press, Buckingham

Fielding R, Wong L, Ko L (1998) Strategies of information disclosure to Chinese cancer patients in an Asian community. *Psychosoc Oncol* **7**: 240–51

Firth S (1997) *Dying, Death and Bereavement in a British Hindu Community*. Peeters, Leuven

Firth S (1999) Hindu widows in Britain: continuity and change. In: Barot R, Bradley H, Fenton S (eds) *Ethnicity, Gender and Social Change*. Macmillan, Basingstoke

Firth S (2001) *Wider Horizons: Care of the Dying in a Multicultural Society*. NCHSPCS, London

Firth S (2004) *Loss, Change and Bereavement in Palliative Care*. Open University Press/McGraw Hill, Maidenhead

Gardner K (1998) Death, burial and bereavement amongst Bengali Muslims. *J Ethn Migr Stud* **24**(3): 507–21

Gardner K (2001) *Age, Narrative and Migration: The Life Course and Life Histories of Bangladeshi Elders in London.* Berg, Oxford

Gilliat-Ray S (2003) Nursing, professionalism, and spirituality. *J Contemp Relig* **18**(3): 335–49

Gunaratnam Y, Bremner I, Pollock L, Weir C (1998) Anti-discrimination, emotions and professional practice. *Eur J Palliat Care* **5**(4): 122–4

Helman C (1994) *Culture, Health and Illness.* Butterworth-Heinemann, Oxford

Henley A, Schott J (1999) *Culture, Religion and Patient Care in a Multiethnic Society.* Age Concern, London

Irish D, Lundquist K, Nelson V (eds) *Ethnic Variations in Dying, Death and Grief: Diversity in Universality.* Taylor and Francis, London

Kakar S (1978) *The Inner World: a Psychoanalytic Study of Childhood and Society in India.* Oxford University Press, Delhi

Kalsi S Singh (1996) Change and continuity in the funeral rituals of Sikhs. In: Howarth G, Jupp P (eds) *Contemporary Issues in the Sociology of Death, Dying and Disposal.* Macmillan, Basingstoke

Kareem J, Littlewood R (eds) (1992) *Intercultural Therapy: Themes, Interpretations and Practice.* Blackwell, Oxford

Krause I (1989) The sinking heart, a Panjabi communication of distress. *Soc Sci Med* **29**(4): 563–75

Kübler-Ross E (1969) *On Death and Dying.* Tavistock, London

Lindemann E (1944) Symptomatology and management of acute grief. *Am J Psychiatry* **101**: 141–8

Leininger M (1996) Response to Cooney article, 'A comparative analysis of transcultural nursing and cultural safety'. *Nurs Prax N Z* **22**(2): 13–15

Morgan JD, Lungani P (eds) (2002) *Death and Bereavement around the World. Vol I: Major Religious Traditions.* Baywood Publishing Co Inc, Amityville, New York

Netto G, Gaag S, Thanki M (2001) *A Suitable Space: Improving Counselling Services for Asian People.* The Policy Press for Joseph Rowntree Foundation, London

Notta II, Warr B (1998) Acorns Children's Hospice, Birmingham. In: Oliviere D, Hargreaves R, Monroe B (eds) *Good Practices in Palliative Care: a Psychosocial Perspective.* Ashgate Arena, Aldershot

Parkes CM (1986) *Bereavement: Studies of Grief in Adult Life.* Penguin, London

Parkes CM, Laungani P, Young B (1997) *Death and Bereavement Across Cultures.* Routledge, London

Parkes CM, Weiss R (1983) *Recovery From Bereavement*. Basic Books, New York

Radcliffe-Brown AR (1964) *The Andaman Islanders*. Free Press, New York

Rosenblatt PC, Walsh R, Jackson (1976) *Grief and Mourning in Cross-cultural Perspectives*. HRAF Press, Washington DC

Seale C (1998) *Constructing Death: the Sociology of Death and Bereavement*. Cambridge University Press, UK

Shoaib K, Peel J (2003) Kashmiri women's perceptions of their emotional and psychological needs, and access to counselling. *Counsell Psychotherap Res* **3**(2): 87–94

Silverman P (2004) Mourning: a changing view. In: Firth P, Luff G, Oliviere D (eds) *Loss, Change and Bereavement in Palliative Care*. Open University Press/Macgraw Hill, Maidenhead

Somerville JE (2001) The experience of informal carers within the Bangladeshi community. *Int J Palliat Care* **7**(5): 240–7

Spruyt O (1999) Community-based palliative care for Bangladeshi patients in East London: accounts of bereaved carers. *Palliat Med* **13**: 119–29

Stroebe M, Schut H (1998) Culture and grief. *Bereavement Care* **17**(1): 7–11

Taylor Mohammed F (2001) Follow fashion monkey never drink good soup: black counsellors and the road to 'inclusion'. *Counsell Psychotherap J* **12**(6): 10–12

Walter T (1999) *On Bereavement*. Open University Press, Buckingham

Wiken U (1988) Bereavement and loss in two Muslim communities: Egypt and Bali compared. *Soc Sci Med* **27**: 451–60

Worden J (1991) *Grief Counselling and Grief Therapy*. 2nd edn. Routledge, London

Glossary

This brief glossary provides an aide memoire of key terms used by South Asians which are not in common usage in the English language

Afsos — a process of giving regrets to the bereaved in all three faiths.

Ahimsa — not to harm or injure any living being, a Hindu philosophy.

Allah — Muslim name for God.

Amrit — literally meaning 'nectar of immortality', it is the sweetened water used during the khalsa initiation ceremony of the Sikhs.

Amrit Sanskar — baptism ceremony for Sikhs.

Arya Samaj — a nineteenth-century Hindu reform movement founded by Swami Dayananda Saraswati, emphasising the Vedic rather than later Brahmanical rituals.

Ashrama — stage of life (for Hindus, there are four).

Asr — mid-afternoon prayer for Muslims.

Assala'mu Alaikum' — an Arabic greeting meaning 'peace be on you'.

Atman — the principle or essence of life (ie. 'soul' for Hindus).

Avatar — an incarnation of God for Hindus, usually of Vishnu, popularly as Rama or Krishna.

Ayurveda — the ancient Vedic science of healing and medicine.

Baisakhi — festival celebrating the creation of the baptism rites for Sikhs.

Bhagavad Gita — a Hindu holy book.

Bhajan — a hymn or a Hindu song.

Bhakti — devotion to a personal God for Sikhs. The Bhakti movement was a religious movement originating in southern India around the sixth century CE that subsequently spread over the next thousand years northward throughout the subcontinent. Although the movement took on its own distinct form, depending on the area it had spread to, the central spiritual practice was the fostering of loving devotion to God.

Bhakti Yoga — the path of devotion for Hindus.

Bhatras — peddlars (a sub-caste of Sikhs).

Bhavan — a place where Hindus elect to go to die.

Bindi — a coloured 'dot' in the middle of the forehead, worn usually by Hindus.

Brahmacharya — student, the first of the four Ashramas for Hindus.

Brahmin — the priestly class or Varna amongst Hindus.

Caste — subdivisions of the four Varnas, based on occupation and ritual purity amongst Hindus and, to a certain extent, amongst Sikhs.

Chamars — a caste of leather workers amongst Sikhs.

Dalits — a modern name for 'untouchables', the lowest of the four Varnas amongst Hindus.

Dasam Granth — collected works of the tenth Sikh Guru.

Dharma — righteousness, morality or virtuous conduct, at personal, family, caste and universal levels for Hundus.

Diva — lighting of a candle by Hindus.

Dukh — a term meaning 'sorrow' or 'sadness', used by all three faiths.

Eid-ul-adha — celebration at the end of the Muslim pilgrimage.

Eid-ul-fitr — celebration at the end of fasting for Muslims.

Ek Onkar — 'There is but one God' (Sikh belief).

Fajr — early morning Muslim prayer.

Fatwa — an edict passed by learned Muslim scholars.

Garuda Purana — Hindu religious scripture.

Granthi — 'Reader' of the Guru Granth Sahib, usually male, whose responsibilities include reading Sikh scriptures, performing ceremonies and the upkeep of the Gurdwara.

Grihasta — Sikh married life.

Grhasthya — householder, the second of the four Ashramas amongst Hindus.

Gurbani — the word of the Guru (or God). The writings of the Gurus and holy Sikh saints as set down in the Guru Granth Sahib.

Gurdwara — 'Doorway to the Guru'. It is the name given to a Sikh place of worship in which the Guru Granth Sahib is installed.

Gurmukhi — from the mouth of the Guru. This is the written form of Punjabi, as standardised by Guru Angad, the second Sikh Guru, used in most of the Sikh religious scripts. It is used today for all modern writing, religious or otherwise.

Guru Granth Sahib — The holy scripture of the Sikhs, containing about 6000 hymns written by six Gurus (First–Fifth, Ninth), and various other Saints from other religions, including Hinduism and Islam. The Sikhs treat the Guru Granth Sahib as a living Guru and thus it is handled with great respect.

Gurpurbs — birthdays of Sikh Gurus.

Guru Nanak — founder of the Sikh religion.

Gutka — a Sikh book of prayers.

Hadith — a collection of actions and sayings of Prophet Muhammad amongst Muslims.

Hajj — Muslim pilgrimage.

Hakims and Pirs — herbalists and faith healers in India.

Halaal — that which is allowed in Islam.

Haraam — that which is forbidden in Islam.

Harimandir — the Golden Temple of Sikhs.

Haumai — an inner egotism and self-centredness present in all human beings that blocks the pathway to enlightenment and union with God.

Havan — a Hindu fire ritual.

Hukam — Divine will or order of God. Hukam can also refer to a passage of the Guru Granth Sahib selected by randomly opening the Sikh scripture during a daily ceremony.

Idat — a period of mourning during which a Muslim woman will not leave her home after the death of her husband.

Ijtihad — a process of deduction from Islamic scriptures.

Imam — a Muslim priest.

Isha — a Muslim prayer late at night.

Jatis — occupational castes for Hindus and Sikhs.

Jats — agriculturists' caste amongst Sikhs.

Jnana (Hindi, gyan) yoga — the path or way of mystical knowledge for Hindus.

Kaaba — a symbol in the middle of the Grand Mosque in Mecca towards which all Muslims in the world turn for praying.

Kanga — comb, one of the five articles of faith that an 'initiated' or Khalsa Sikh must wear. It also symbolises a disciplined and hygienic lifestyle.

Kara — steel circular bracelet, one of the five articles of faith that an 'initiated' or Khalsa Sikh must wear. It symbolises God's infinity, a circle having no beginning or end.

Karma — action. The Hindu law of karma is cause and effect; good thoughts and deeds have good results, negative ones have bad consequences. They carry over into the next life, and keep the wheel of reincarnation going.

Karma yoga — the path of action through ritual and sacrifices for Hindus.

Kaur — literally 'princess'. The middle or last name given to all female Sikhs.

Kes-dhari — non-baptised Sikh.

Kesh — uncut hair, one of the five articles of faith that an 'initiated' or Khalsa Sikh must keep. It symbolises spirituality and many Sikhs believe it is an aid to increasing spiritual energy. It also signifies the acceptance of the natural form God gave to humanity, as well as giving Sikhs a unique identity.

Khalsa — fraternity of the pure. Khalsa Sikhs are a community of Sikhs that have undergone the Sikh initiation ceremony (pahul). Khalsa Sikhs are required to wear the five symbols of the Sikh faith at all times, and live by a strict code of conduct that requires, amongst other things, daily meditation, vegetarianism and a ban on taking any form of intoxicants. Khalsa Sikhs constitute the orthodoxy within Sikhism and will lead all religious functions and ceremonies.

Khanda — a Sikh symbol. The two swords symbolise fighting for what is right, the circle portraying that there is no beginning or end to God.

Kirpan — a ceremonial short sword and one of the five articles of faith that an 'initiated' or or Khalsa Sikh must keep.

Kismat/qismat — 'fate, destiny' (Urdu).

Krishna — a Hindu God.

Kshatrya — warriors and rulers/kings: the second Varna amongst Hindus.

Kshera — a pair of knee-length shorts, one of the five articles of faith that an 'initiated' or Khalsa Sikh must wear. It is a symbol of high moral character and self-control.

Langar — free community kitchen found in all Sikh Gurdwaras, which provides free meals and is open to all people regardless of caste, colour or creed. The langar is an integral part of the Sikh religion and is a potent symbol of the social and spiritual equality taught by the Sikh Gurus.

Maghrib — evening prayer for Muslims.

Meenakshi or **mata-ji** — female energy (a Hindu godess).

Miri-Piri — concept of the Guru having spiritual authority (piri) and also assuming a temporal role (miri). The sixth Sikh Guru, Guru Hargobind Ji, exemplified this by wearing two swords.

Moksha (or **mukti**) — spiritual liberation from the cycle of birth, death and rebirth.

Mona Sikhs — Sikhs who retain their affiliation to their religion but remove all outward symbols of Sikhism.

Naam — the divine Name or essence of God that pervades all creation: a Sikh belief.

Naam Simran — the devotional practice of meditating on the divine Name. This is the core form of Sikh worship.

Nirankar — 'formless'; one of the many names for God used in Sikhism.

Om, Aum — a sacred Hindu syllable, symbolising the beginning and the end, and all creation.

Pahul — the administration of amrit during the Khalsa initiation ceremony for Sikhs.

Puja — Hindu prayers.

Qur'an — the Muslim holy book.

Radha — a Hindu goddess.

Rahiras — the holy path (a Sikh recitation).

Ram — a Hindu God.

Ramgarhias — craftsman (a Sikh sub-caste).

Sabr —an Arabic word meaning 'unconditional contentment with the Divine': words used by Muslims during bereavement.

Sahaj — union with the supreme reality for Sikhs.

Sakrat — the final rite of giving a Muslim holy water during final gasps whilst the shahadah is recited.

Salah — a Muslim prayer.

Sampradaya — 'sect'; a religious organisation associated with a Guru (teacher).

Samsara — the cycle of birth, death and rebirth for Sikhs and Hindus.

Sanatan(a) Dharma — a term used by many Hindus to describe their religion: the eternal religion.

Sangat — a fellowship of Sikh believers.

Sannyasi — ascetic or holy man, the fourth Ashrama amongst Hindus.

Sanskrit — an ancient language akin to Latin.

Sari — a form of Asian dress.

Sati — a custom of burning Hindu widows with their husbands.

Sawm — fasting for Muslims.

Shahadah — the main tenet for Muslims in the belief in one and only God with Muhammed as his final messenger.

Shalwar kameez — a form of Asian dress, particularly for Muslims.

Shariah — Islamic law.

Shishya — a Sanskrit word meaning 'disciple'.

Shiva — a Hindu God.

Shraddha — Hindu postmortem rites for ten to thirty days following cremation, and annually.

Shudra — peasants and labourers: the fourth of the four Varnas amongst Hindus.

Singh — literally means 'lion'. The middle or last name given to all male Sikhs.

Sita — a Hindu goddess.

Sohilla — a Sikh prayer.

Sufism — a branch of Islamic beliefs.

Sukh — happiness.

Sunnah — that which should be emulated by Muslims and was practiced by Prophet Muhammad.

Swaminarayan — a nineteenth-century Hindu reformer.

Tawiz — a black string containing religious Muslim scriptures, worn around the neck or wrist.

Topi — skull cap.

Tulsi — a sacred leaf (of a basil type) used to purify the dying Hindu.

Ulemas — learned Islamic scholars.

Upanishads — a group of Hindu religious texts.

Vaishya — merchants, farmers, the third Varna for Hindus.

Vanaprastha — forest dweller, the third Ashrama for Hindus.

Varna — denotes colour. The four great Hindu social classes described in Vedic literature (circa 1500 BC).

Varnashramadharma — another term for Hinduism, encompassing the four Varnas, Ashramas and dharma.

Vishnu — a Hindu God.

Vishnuvites — followers of Vishnu, a Hindu God.

Waheguru — 'wonderful Lord', recited when a Sikh dies.

Wudu — ablution for Muslims before prayers.

Zakah — monies that have to be given to the poor by Muslims as a religious obligation.

Zam Zam — holy water for Muslims.

Zuhr — a prayer around midday.

Agencies working with South-Asian communities

Sally Killian

Afiya Trust, 27-29 Vauxhall Grove, London SW8 1SY, UK
Tel 020 7582 0434, fax 020 7582 2552, www.afiya-trust.org

African Caribbean Leukaemia Trust, PO Box 670, Croydon CR9 5DP, UK
Tel 020 8667 1122, fax 020 8667 1626, email info@aclt.org, www.aclt.org

Asian Cancer Information Project, Greenwich & Bexley Primary Care Trust,
221 Erith Road, Bexley Heath, Kent DA7 6HZ, UK
Tel 020 8298 6276, fax 020 8298 6049

Bradford Cancer Support Centre, Daisy Bank, Bradford BD9 6RN, UK
Tel 01274 777711 / 776688, fax 01274 776555

Breast Cancer Care, 210 New King's Road, London SW6 4NZ, UK
Tel 020 7384 4604, fax 020 7394 3387, www.breastcancercare.org.uk

Bridges Project, Murrayhall Community Trust, Neptune Health Park,
Sedgley Road West, Tipton DY4 8LU, UK
Tel 0121 607 6404, fax 0121 607 6403, murrayhall@which.net

Cancer BACUP, 3 Bath Place, Rivington Street, London EC2A 3JR, UK
Tel 020 7920 7210, fax 020 7696 9002, www.cancerbacup.org.uk

Cancer BACUP Information Centre (Help Advocacy Service),
St Bartholomew's Hospital, First Floor, King George V Wing,
London EC1A 7BE, UK
Tel 020 7601 7092, fax 020 7601 7893

Cancer Black Care, 112 Denmark Hill, Camberwell, London SE5 8RX, UK
Tel 020 7501 8787, fax 020 7501 8686, www.cancerblackcare.org

Cancer Black Care (Manchester), 464 Chester Road, Old Trafford, Manchester
M16 9HE, UK
Tel 0845 4504247, email info@blackhealthagency.org.uk
www.blackhealthagency.org.uk

Cancer Information Centre, Health Shop, Homerton University Hospital,
Homerton Row, London E9 6SR, UK
Tel 020 8510 5191

Cancer Information & Support Services, Walsall tPCT, The Hatherton
Centre, Challenge Building, Hatherton Road, Walsall WS1 1YB, UK
Tel 0800 783 9050 (freephone), fax 01922 858986
email cissenquiries@walsall.nhs.uk

Cancer You Are Not Alone (CYANA), 31 Snowhill Road, Manor Park,
London E12 6BE, UK
Tel 020 8553 5366, fax 020 8553 5366, email cyana@supanet.com
www.cyana.org

CLIC Sargent Cancer Care, 118 Gatley Road, Cheshire SK8 4AD, UK
Tel 0161 610 7150, fax 0161 491 5107

Compton Hospice, 4 Compton Road West, Wolverhampton WV3 9DH, UK
Tel 01902 774500 (ext 232), fax 01902 745232

Connexions, Direct Information & Advice for Young People
Tel 080 800 13 2 19, www.connexions-direct.com

Coping with Cancer Centre, Helen Webb House, 35 Westleigh Road, Leicester
LE3 0HH, UK
Tel 0116 223 0055, language line (South-Asian languages) 0116 223 0020,
fax 0116 223 0062, email post@c-w-c.org.uk, www.c-w-c.org.uk

Derby Cancer Centre, Junction 11, Derbyshire Royal Infirmary, London Road,
Derby DE1 2QY, UK
Tel 01332 347141 (ext 4038)

Directory of Cancer Information, Available in BME Languages, Cancer
Equality, Unit 18, Boardman House, 64 Broadway, London E15 1NT, UK
Tel 020 8432 0565, fax 020 8432 0569, email info@cancerequality.org.uk

Enfield Disability Action, CancerLIFE, Community House, 311 Fore Street, Edmonton, London N9 0PZ, UK
Tel 020 8373 6222, fax 020 8373 6223, email can@eda.demon.co.uk, www.eda.demon.co.uk

Janki Foundation for Global Healthcare, Research/awareness of spirituality and health, 449–451 High Road, London NW10 2JJ, UK
Tel 020 8459 1400/9090, fax 020 8459 9091, email values@jankifoundation.org www.jankifoundation.org

Learning & Skills Council
Tel 0870 900 6800, email info@lsc.gov.uk, www.lsc.gov.uk

Macmillan Cancer Information & Support Centre, Central Outpatients Department, University Hospital of North Staffordshire, Hartshill Road, Stoke on Trent ST4 7PA, UK
Tel 01782 554363, fax 01782 555334

Macmillan Cancer Relief Cancer Voices Project, Macmillan Cancerlink, Cancer Voices Project, 89 Albert Embankment, London SE1 7UQ, UK
Tel 020 7091 2004, fax 020 7840 7841

Macmillan Palliative Care Team, King Edward VII Hospital, St Leonards Road, Windsor, Berkshire SL4 3DP, UK
Tel 01753 863 960, fax 01753 636139

Medway Maritime Hospital, Windmill Road, Gillingham, Kent ME7 5NY, UK
Tel 01634 825288, fax 01634 825210

National Cancer Alliance, PO Box 579, Oxford OX4 1LB, UK
www.temworkfile.org.uk

Newham General Hospital, Cancer Services, Glen Road, Plaistow, London E13 8SL, UK
Tel 020 7363 8393, fax 020 7363 8262

Policy & Research Institute of Ageing & Ethnicity (PRIAE), 31–32 Park Row, Leeds LS1 5JD, UK
Tel 0113 285 5990, fax 0113 285 5999, email info@priae.org, www.priac.org

Rotherham Hospice, Broom Road, Rotherham S60 2SW, UK
Tel 01709 829900, fax 01709 371702

The Courtyard Information Centre, Sandwell General Hospital, Lyndon, West Bromwich B71 4HJ, UK
Tel 0121 607 7972

The Multicultural Health Resource & Information Centre, Butetown Health Centre, Loudon Square, Cardiff CF1 5HZ, Wales, UK

The National Cancer Alliance, Leicester Charity Link, 20A Millstone Lane, Leicester LE1 5JN, UK
Tel 0116 222 2202, fax 0116 222 2201

Trent Palliative Care Centre, Sykes House, Little Common Lane (off Abbey Lane), Sheffield S11 2EN, UK
Tel 0114 262 0174, fax 0114 236 2916, www.riprap.org.uk

Umeed Asian Women's Project, Beaument Street, Sneinton, Nottingham NG2 4PJ, UK
Tel 0115 958 6959, fax 0115 924 2595

Wandsworth Cancer Resource Centre, 20–22 York Road, Battersea, London SW11 3QE, UK
Tel 020 7978 6203, fax 020 7978 6505

INDEX

11th September 2001 ('9/11'), attack on
New York City 163
7th July 2005 ('7/7'), attack on London,
UK 163

A

acculturation 31, 39, 69, 72, 119, 169
Acorns Children's Hospices 51, 117–20,
123, 125, 127, 128, 162, 178, 181
adolescence 132, 135, 136, 140, 144
'Africanisation' (political policy of) 60
AIDS 40, 133, 174
alcoholics 17
Allah 34
analgesia 37, 46, 149, 150, 152
anger 140, 141, 149, 151, 152, 171
anxiety 48, 49, 61, 114, 120, 121, 126,
149, 152, 175
Ashramas 58
Asian Liaison Officer 120
Asian Mother Support Group 120
Asr 35
Association for Children with Life
Threatening and Terminal
Conditions (ACT) 118, 132
asylum seekers 177
Ayurvedic medicine 65

B

'bad death' 62, 63, 65, 72, 75, 77
befrienders 124
bereavement 5, 8, 40, 50, 53, 54, 59,
76–9, 82, 99, 110, 117, 126, 129,
159, 167, 174–80
bereavement support 78, 110, 174, 175,
177–9
Bhagavad Gita 57, 59, 62, 67, 69, 70,
75–7
Bindi 30
black counsellors 175, 182

Brahmins 58, 60
burials 49, 50

C

Caldicott Guardianship 162
cancer 4–7, 10, 18, 42, 54, 64, 67, 72, 73,
79, 81, 103–6, 108–12, 115, 118,
130, 133, 135, 139, 145, 147, 148,
152, 174, 180
Cancer Plan, The (NHS) 3–5
caste 57–60, 70, 71, 76, 84, 86, 89, 91, 92
Census (2001) 11, 12, 25, 34, 40, 68,
124, 130
Children Act, The (1989) 133
Christian chaplains 34, 160, 161
Church of England 155, 161
Church Times, The 155
cinema visits 142
cleanliness 35, 36, 38
Commission for Racial Equality 103
community workers 104, 106, 119
Compton Hospice 178
confidentiality 44, 134, 143, 162, 174,
176, 177
Connexions Service 137–9
coronary heart disease (CHD) 72
coroners 178
counselling 47, 55, 122, 139, 167, 175–8,
180, 182
cremation 61, 76, 77, 80, 98, 167
Creutzfeldt-Jakob disease (CJD) 133
cultural competence 13, 16–19, 21, 22,
69, 175
cultural taboos 104, 106

D

Dalits 58
dance 105, 109, 113
death rites 47, 61
dehumanisation 18
depression 130, 140, 171

Dharma 57, 58, 59, 66
diabetes 5, 6, 9, 19, 42, 72
diamorphine 148, 149
Disability Discrimination Act, The (1995) 138
disclosure 43, 44, 57, 64, 66, 67, 73, 120, 121, 180
Diva 30
diversity 6, 9, 11–17, 20–2, 51, 93, 99, 113, 143, 158, 164, 175, 179, 180
diversity management 13, 15–17, 21, 22
DJ project 108
doctrine of double effect 37, 149, 153
drawing 105, 167
Duchenne muscular dystrophy 133, 140, 141, 174

E

end of life care 7, 100
euthanasia 37, 38, 45, 64–7, 92

F

Fajr 35
Family Law Act, The (1969) 132
family structures 126, 168, 169
Fatwa 36, 49
fentanyl 148
Florence Nightingale 11

G

Gandhi, Mohandas 'Mahatma' 65, 66
Ganges (river) 62, 63, 74, 76, 77, 173
Garuda Purana 62, 67
gender roles 38, 176
General Medical Council, UK (GMC) 147, 152
genetic disorders 42
genetic engineering 92, 93
Gillick competence 133
Gold Standards Framework (GSF) 4, 8
'good death' 57, 62, 63, 66, 67, 69, 72, 73, 76, 129, 173
    (see also 'bad death')
grief 44, 50, 69, 77, 125, 169, 170–2, 176, 179, 180–2

guilt 50, 61, 64, 171
Gurdwara 91, 97
Guru Granth Sahib 83–91, 93, 97, 99

H

Hadith 36
Hajj 35
Halal 36, 37
Haram 36, 37
Health Service Journal, The 156
Help the Aged 9
HIV 40, 133
holistic care 69, 131, 158, 162, 167
Hospital Chaplaincies Council 155
Human Rights Act, The (1998) 162

I

identity 11, 31, 57, 86, 126, 135, 136, 140, 168, 169
Ijtihad 36, 40
imam 158
incense 53, 74, 76
incontinence 75
institutional racism 13, 14, 17, 19
Isha 35
Islamophobia 163

J

Jesus 34, 83, 84
Job (Book of) 174
joss sticks 30
Judeo-Christian traditions 29, 34
Judgement Day 43

K

Kanga 86, 96
Kara 30, 86, 96
Karma 57–9, 66, 71, 75, 76, 83, 98, 171
Katchera 96
Kesh 86, 96
Khanda 96
King's Fund 116, 178
Kirpan 86, 96
Krishna 59, 60–2, 83
Kshatriyas 58

L

Learning and Skills Council, The 137, 138
leukaemia 42, 132
levomepromazine 149
life-limiting illness 117, 120, 125, 127, 135, 136
Liverpool Care of the Dying Pathway 7

M

Macmillan Gold Standard Framework 7
Macmillan nurses 108, 109
Maghrib 35
magnetic resonance imaging (MRI) 48
Mecca 7, 35, 38, 45–7, 49, 53
microcephaly 132
modesty 39, 52, 74, 96
Moksha 59, 71, 83, 89
mourning 50, 59, 61, 62, 77, 99, 168, 169, 171, 172
multi-faith chaplaincy 156, 158, 163–5
Multi-Faith Group for Healthcare Chaplaincy 159
music 105, 109, 141
Muslim Bereavement Service 178

N

Naam Simran 89, 90
Nanak 83–6, 88–90, 93, 100
National Carers Strategy 3
National Council for Hospice and Specialist Palliative Care Services 23, 54, 81, 116, 118
National Institute for Clinical Excellence (NICE) 3, 4, 6
neuromuscular disorders 42
New Opportunities Fund 78, 105

O

oil lamps 74
oncology 3, 113
opiates 74, 131
opioids 46, 75, 147, 150
organ transplantation 49

P

painting 106
Palliative Care Service Guidelines (2003) 132
Parekh Report, The 155, 165
Patient's Charter, The (1991) 159
peripheral vascular disease 19
poetry 104, 105
poor English (language) 167
post-mortems 48, 76, 98, 178
poverty 17, 18, 167, 174
prayer beads 30, 74, 97
Preferred Place of Care (PPC) 7
premature death 133, 169
promiscuity 39
Prophet Muhammad 34, 36, 43, 44, 46
Protection from Harassment Act, The (1997) 14
psychological support 5, 69, 122, 124

Q

Qur'an 34, 36, 38, 40, 41, 44, 46, 48, 49, 53, 172

R

Race Relations Amendment Act, The (2001) 20
racial harassment 14
racism 13, 14, 17–19, 163, 171
radiotherapy 148
Rama 59
Ramadan 35
reflective practice 148
refugees 168
reincarnation 71, 98, 99
Royal College of Nursing (RCN) 142, 145
Royal College of Paediatrics and Child Health (RCPCH) 118, 128, 131

S

Sabr 50
Sakrat 46, 173
Salah 34, 35

salvation 59, 83, 84, 86, 87, 89, 90, 171
Sampradaya 60
Samsara 59, 62, 71, 83
Sandwell and Dudley Cruse Bereavement
      Centre 178
Sanskrit 58, 70, 84
Sawm 35
sedation 149
Select Committee Inquiry into Palliative
      Care 143
self-awareness 16, 17, 19, 22, 79, 148
Shahadah 34, 46, 150
Shariah 35, 37, 49, 54
Shi'a tradition 36
Shiva 59, 61
shrouding 48
Shudras 58
socio-economic status 168
South Asian Palliative Care Arts Aware-
      ness Project (SAPCAA) 78, 105
Special Educational Needs 123, 138, 144
stem-cell research 92, 93
stereotypes 18, 127, 147, 179
storytelling 105
Strategic Health Authority, The 13, 24,
      137
structured reflection 148
substance-abusers 17
Sufism 84
suicide 37, 45, 65, 66
Sunni tradition 36
symptom-management 132, 148, 150

T

Tawiz 30, 46
Topi 30
traditional healers 45, 74
transitional journeys 139–41
tuberculosis 64
turban 30, 88, 92, 96, 172
tyrosinaemia 132

U

Upanishads 59

V

Vaishyas 58
Varna 57
vegetarian diet/food 72, 91
Vishnu 30, 59, 60, 70
vomiting 75

W

withdrawing treatment 47
Women's Royal Voluntary Service
      (WRVS) 157
wudu 38

Y

yoga 59, 62
Young Adults' Transition Project —
      Optimum Health Services
      (NHS, 1999) 138

Z

Zakah 35
Zam Zam 46
Zuhr 35

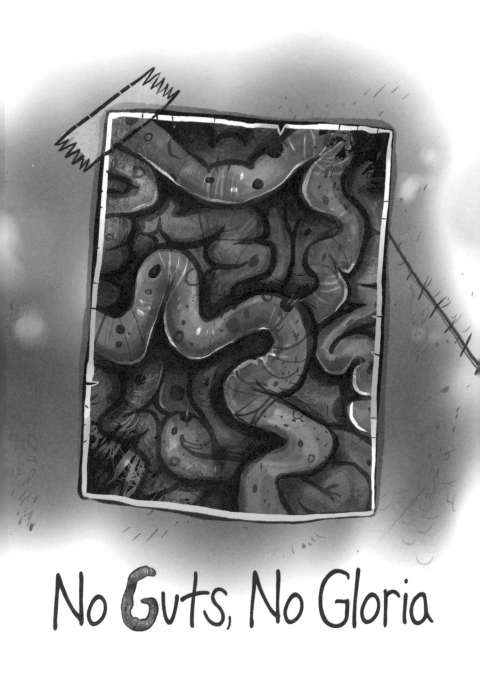

No Guts, No Gloria

Chapter 1

Dear Future Me,

I hope everything's going great for you (meaning me) whenever you're reading this. Because right now, your (my) life has been nothing but crazy since I found Dr Frankenstein's journal!

If you've forgotten, there were two journals. Mine (this one) that I wrote everything down in so I would never forget everything that's happened.

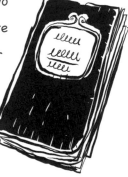

I only had a few pages of Dr Frankenstein's journal.

EEEK!

Like the ones where Frankenstein described where he found his monster's brain, eyeballs and butt. I may not have had all the pages, but I definitely had the most disgusting ones! But while they did have lots of nasty stuff in them, they didn't seem to have a lot of clues.

Clues I needed to save my family.

It was still strange to think that I had a big family out there ... somewhere. Not that long ago I was living in Shelley's Orphanage for Lost and Neglected Children. Back then, I didn't think I had any family at all. It wasn't until the orphanage closed down that I found Dr Frankenstein's journal.

I also found out that I was the son of Frankenstein's monster! I have to admit – that did freak me out.

It also explained why one of my eyes is blue and the other green. Why one of my hands is much bigger than the other. And why my legs are two different sizes.

Body parts from lots of people went into making my dad. And he had passed down all of their legs, feet, eyes and hands to me.

All of those people whose parts went into my dad probably had relatives who were still alive. I was related to them too. They were like my cousins!

Cousins I had to find – and fast!

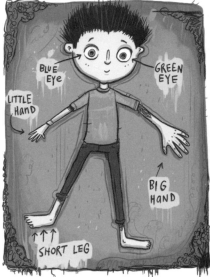

Because if I didn't, Fran Kenstein would get to them first. Fran was the daughter of Dr Frankenstein, and she had stolen her dad's journal from me (luckily, I had copies of a few of the pages).

With the info she had from Dr F's journal, Fran planned to use my cousins to make a new monster.

I didn't have anything against monsters.
I mean, my dad was one. I had never
met him, but I assumed he was a
decent person.

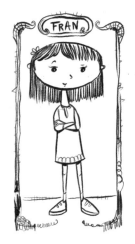

But when I said that Fran planned to
use my cousins, what I meant was that
she planned to take a hand from one, a
leg from another and so on.

I couldn't let that happen to my family (even if I
didn't know who they were). Which meant I had to
warn my cousins before Fran could get to them.

But to warn them, I had to find them. That meant
figuring out the clues in the pages I did have from
Dr Frankenstein's journal – like this one, about the
Monster's large intestine.

As I said, I may not have had all the pages, but I
definitely had the most disgusting ones. This one was
full of horrible pictures, but it didn't have much in the
way of clues.

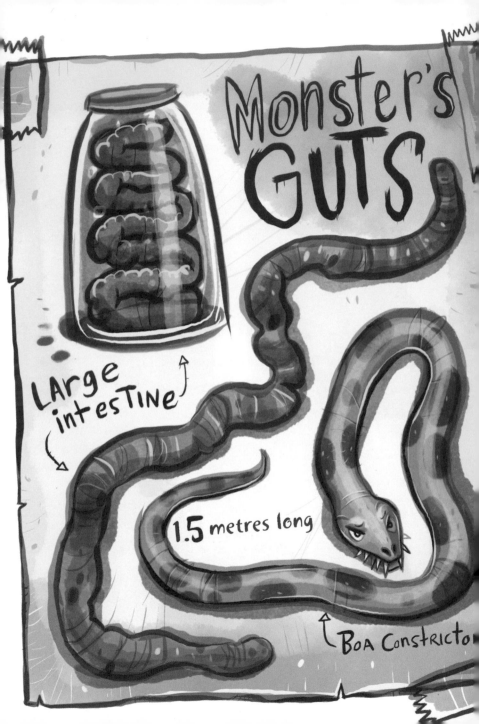

In fact, it only had a few words on it: "Large intestine" and "Monster's Guts". And seeing as "guts" is just another word for large intestine, that didn't really tell me anything at all.

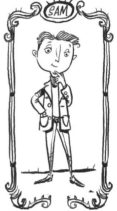

Of course, that wouldn't have stopped Sam.

Sam was my second cousin (the second cousin I had found, that is). His dad was a famous private eye whose actual eye had gone into my dad. Which is pretty disgusting, but also pretty cool. Because that's what made Sam related to me.

Sam was a police detective in Los Angeles. He'd know where to find clues in Dr F's journal.

But Sam was still busy wrapping up the case I had helped him to solve. Which I totally understood. (If you don't remember why it was so important that the man we caught stay behind bars, just read the last part of my journal).

Sam didn't even have time to say goodbye. Instead, he gave me something:

My dad's police file from the Los Angeles Police Department Monster Crimes Unit!

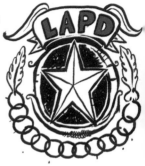

I left the LAPD headquarters, looking for a place to read the file. I found the local library and sat down at a table.

I hoped my dad's file would help me to solve the other big mystery in my life: what had happened to him? Where did my dad go after he dropped me off at the orphanage and disappeared?

I may have had the eye of a detective, just like Sam, but I couldn't solve this mystery.

I studied the police file from front to back. There was some stuff about my dad from before I was born (No crimes, though. I suppose he was a pretty decent person). But there was nothing in the file from after I was born.

Still, I hoped there might be some clue about where my dad was now. So my eyes lit up when I saw this:

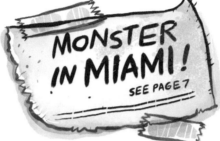

When I saw that headline, I got excited.

Until I read the article. The monster in it wasn't my dad. It was the Vampire.

Sam once told me, "Just because a clue doesn't tell you everything, doesn't mean it's telling you nothing."

Maybe that was true. But this wasn't even a clue. It was just an old newspaper article that had been put in the wrong Monster Crimes Unit file.

Still, I knew Sam wouldn't just throw the article away. He'd look again to see if there was anything useful in it.

So I took another look. And that's when I saw it!

Under the photo, it said that the Vampire's bodyguard was nicknamed "The Monster's Guts" – because he was brave and he protected a monster.

I flipped back through the pages I had from Dr Frankenstein's journal. On the page describing the large intestine, it also said "The Monster's Guts".

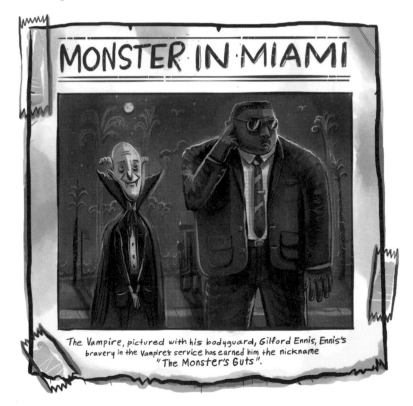

MONSTER IN MIAMI

The Vampire, pictured with his bodyguard, Gilford Ennis, Ennis's bravery in the Vampire's service has earned him the nickname "The Monster's Guts".

Maybe Dr Frankenstein hadn't written that as another way of saying "my monster's large intestine". Perhaps it was the nickname of the man the intestine had come from!

That had to be it! That meant the article wasn't misfiled. It had been put in there because my dad got his large intestine from a man who was the Vampire's bodyguard!

I just might have found out where my dad got his guts!

Even better, I thought there was a chance the bodyguard might still be alive. I didn't know much about science or medicine (or a lot of things, really). But I did know that everyone has a large AND a small intestine. You don't need both, right?

Even if my medical knowledge was wrong, I knew the Vampire was still alive. Or, not alive, but undead or whatever. If a man like that had kicked the bucket, it would definitely make the news. But I didn't find anything more about the Vampire on the internet.

Except his email address!

So I sent him an email. And he wrote back!

I had a lead about another cousin! Maybe I really did have the eye of a detective.

And the guts of a professional bodyguard!

From: Vamp@Ipingvillage.com

Re: A question about "The Monster's Guts"

Dear sir,

Thank you for your email enquiry. Your suspicions are correct. I would be glad to tell you more in person if you would care to visit me at my home.

Yours,

The Vampire

Chapter 2

A day later, I was in Florida.

The Vampire's email had included a plane ticket. What wasn't included were answers to any of my questions about his bodyguard. He just said we would talk when I met him at his home.

That turned out to be in a place called Iping Village. It was a retirement community near Miami, Florida.

The security guard opened the front gate for me. "I bet you're here to see your grandparents," he said. "Go right in!"

I told him I was actually there to meet a cousin, who was related to me through my dad's large intestine.

The guard looked at me as though I was crazy.

The Vampire had emailed me the address of his house. So I started looking for it.

Iping Village was right by the beach, with lots of little houses on a golf course. Every few metres there were kiosks with posters and signs stuck on them.

All of them had signs advertising a show that was playing tonight:

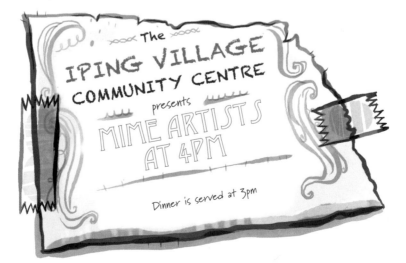

The
IPING VILLAGE
COMMUNITY CENTRE
presents
MIME ARTISTS
AT 4PM

Dinner is served at 3pm

Who wants to see mime artists? At four in the afternoon? Or eat dinner at three?

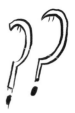

As I walked to the Vampire's house, I saw the answer: old people.

Iping Village was full of them. Riding on golf carts. Slowly. Very slowly. Or walking – even more slowly – with four-pronged walking sticks.

That's when I had a horrifying thought.

I had been wondering why the Vampire wanted to live in the sunniest place in the entire United States.

Suddenly, it all made sense. All these old people were easy pickings!

I mean, they couldn't move very fast (even on golf carts, their max speed was fifteen miles per hour).

Not to mention, in a place where the average age looked to be ninety years old, it was only natural that some people passed away every year.

If the Vampire got to a few of them early, who would notice?

Then I had an even more terrible thought: why did the Vampire invite me here instead of answering my questions over email? Was it because he was tired of only drinking old people and wanted some fresh blood?! YUCK!

Despite the hot Florida sun, a shiver went down my spine. I didn't want to believe a cousin of mine would work for someone as evil as that.

But even if that made my cousin evil, too, he didn't deserve what Fran Kenstein had in store for him. I had to warn him.

Without the Vampire getting his fangs into me!

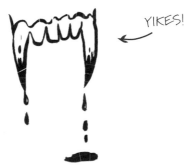
YIKES!

The question was – how was I going to do that?

I had reached the door of the Vampire's house. As I stood there trying to think, a dog lying outside started barking at me.

It was an old dog. It barely lifted its head to let out a...

Woof Woof!

"Hey there," I whispered. "Shhh! I'm trying to work out how to warn my cousin who I'm related to through his large intestine without being sucked dry by the Vampire!"

It gave me the same look the security guard had. And kept barking.

I had to do something to make it stop barking. I closed my eyes and tried to think of what to do.

Only to have someone rush up and tackle me to the ground!

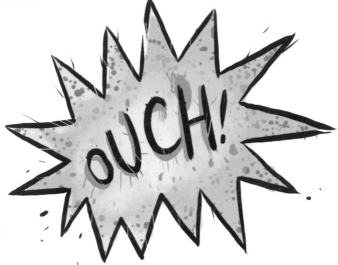

Chapter 3

OOMPH! I hit the ground hard. Holding me down was a woman who was about twenty. Or thirty. It was hard to tell with her hand pushing my face down.

"Why are you lurking outside the Vampire's house?" she asked.

"MRRRMPH," I replied. I was trying to say, "Please don't feed me to the Vampire!" But it was hard to talk with her hand over my mouth.

She took her hand off my mouth. "What do you want with the Vampire?" she asked.

"He invited me here! My name's JD! I just want to talk to him," I cried, "about his bodyguard."

As proof, I pointed to my journal, which had fallen out of my back pocket. The newspaper article about the Vampire's bodyguard was sticking out of it.

"I'm the Vampire's bodyguard," said the woman as she got off of me. The dog hadn't moved but continued to bark at me.

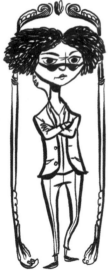

The woman took my journal and looked at the picture. I looked at it, too. And then at the woman who had tackled me.

"You're the Vampire's bodyguard? You look a little shorter now," I said. "And also more like a girl. And also can you get this dog to stop barking? And also ... didn't the Vampire tell you I was coming?!"

As she studied the picture, she told the dog, "Good boy, Renfield. This is JD."

The dog stopped barking immediately.

"Renfield is the Vampire's dog," the woman explained. "He doesn't move much, but he's an excellent guard dog. I trained him to bark at anyone he's never seen before. Now that he's met you, JD, he'll never bark at you again."

Then she turned to me. "And yes, the Vampire did say you were coming. But you're not what I was expecting. You have to admit, you do look a bit peculiar."

I nodded. When you have one blue eye and one green, and one hand a lot bigger than the other, you get that a lot.

"Well, anyway, I'm okay," I said, getting to my feet. "I suppose it was just a mix-up. No need to apologize."

"You're right," she replied. "That's why I didn't apologize. A bodyguard has to assess every potential risk to her client and act accordingly. I acted accordingly."

She looked at the newspaper photograph of the Vampire and his bodyguard.

"That's my father in the picture," she said. "He was the Vampire's bodyguard. I've got the job now. My name's Gloria."

As she looked at her dad's face in the photo, her mouth turned very slightly at the corners. It took me a second to recognize what her mouth was doing. She was smiling. By the time I worked it out, the tiny smile was gone.

Instead, she was staring at me. Suspiciously.

"And seeing as I'm his bodyguard now," she said coldly, "it's my job to ask: why are you curious about the Vampire's security?"

I told her my whole story, including how Fran Kenstein would be after her because she was my cousin.

I must have talked for at least ten minutes!

She listened carefully the whole time, concentrating on every word.

Finally, when I had finished, she said, "Okay, got it."

That wasn't exactly the reaction I was expecting. I thought she'd be surprised to hear about me, my dad and Fran Kenstein.

It's not exactly your typical fourteen-year-old's life story.

Not to mention, a big part of that story was how her father's guts ended up in my dad!

"I'm sorry to have to tell you about that," I said. "I mean, it's not as though it was my fault. Or my dad's fault. But still..."

"Don't apologize. You had to tell me that so I could adequately assess the risk Fran Kenstein poses. A bodyguard needs to know the risks to do her job," Gloria said.

"I am not happy to hear about what happened to my father after he died," she said in a tone of voice that didn't sound sad. Or happy. It was all business. "But I don't have time to be sad right now. I have a job to do. The same job my family has always done: keep the Vampire safe while he sleeps during the day like he's doing now."

"That's your family's job?" I asked, confused.

"Protecting the Vampire has always been my family's responsibility," Gloria explained. "In fact, only someone in my family can do it."

"I don't understand," I said.

"Most people don't," she said, handing me a business card. "But a bodyguard doesn't have time to stand around answering everyone's questions about the rules the Vampire lives by. So I made this."

The top of the card read "Vampire FAQ". Below that were all sorts of questions and answers about the Vampire:

Vampire FAQ
(Frequently Annoying Questions)

- Can the Vampire enter a house without being invited?

  Unless it's your own home, entering a house without being invited is breaking and entering. No one can do that without breaking the law. That includes the Vampire.

- When can the Vampire go outside?

  The Vampire can <u>ONLY</u> go out at night. He will explode if he goes out in the sun.

- So can he go outside on a cloudy day?

  No.

- How about a rainy, cloudy day?

  No!

- How about a day that's –

  NO! He can <u>ONLY</u> go out after sunset.

- Why are your family members the only ones who can look after the Vampire?

  The Vampire can only make a pact with one family to be his bodyguards. No one else can protect him.

- Yes, but why is that?

  <u>Because that's the RULE.</u>

- But what would happen if someone else tries to protect him?

  I don't even want to know the answer to that. So, trust me – if I don't want to know, you don't want to know.

"No one else can protect the Vampire while he sleeps but a member of my family," said Gloria. "My grandfather protected the Vampire. When my grandfather died, my dad became the Vampire's bodyguard."

"When he died, it became my job," said Gloria. "And it's a dangerous job — the Vampire has made a few enemies in the past four hundred years. One in particular."

Gloria looked around.

"Who are you looking for?" I asked.

"No one," she replied. "You can't look for someone you can't see."

I had no idea what that meant. But before I could ask, she turned and looked into my eye (the green one).

"You came here to warn me about the threat posed to my person by Ms Kenstein," she said. "And you've done that. So please go. I can't afford any distractions while I'm on duty."

She was too busy looking around to even look at me when she said the words.

I didn't know what to say either. Every other cousin I had found had been pleased to meet me.

But I suppose I had to expect that not all of them would be like that. Still, I had only found three relatives so far. The fact that one wanted me to get lost was pretty disappointing.

Okay, more than disappointing. But nevermind. I had a lot more cousins to find and warn about Fran. I had already told Gloria everything she needed to know. Besides, it seemed as though she could take care of herself. It wasn't as though she needed my help. She had definitely made that clear.

So I said goodbye and headed off to find more cousins who actually wanted me around.

On my way out of Iping Village, I walked across the golf course.

There was one of those kiosks with a poster for the mime show. It was shady underneath it. Renfield had found his way there (I suppose he could move, just really slowly) and was resting in a cool spot.

There was no one else around. It seemed as though all the other old people here were like the Vampire and enjoyed taking a long nap during the day.

So I sat there next to Renfield to write down what had happened in my journal.

But as soon as I started, Renfield barked. And barked. It couldn't have been because of me. Gloria had said that Renfield was trained to bark at people he hadn't seen before. But he had already met me.

So I looked up from my journal to find out why Renfield was barking. And saw...

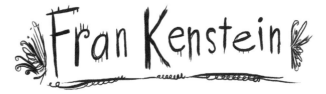

Chapter 4

I stared at Fran Kenstein across the eighth hole of the Iping Village golf course.

How could she be here?! She didn't have my dad's police file, and that's what had led me to Gloria.

Apparently, she had the same question for me.

"How are you here?!" asked Fran. "How could you have found out about Gloria before me – when only I have access to all of Dr Frankenstein's journal?"

That was true. Fran did have all the pages of her father's journal.

But only because she had stolen them from me!

"I suppose I shouldn't be surprised," said Fran. "You've already inconvenienced me twice. I thought that framing you and having you arrested would get you out of the way. Apparently not."

She smiled. Which worried me. Anything that made Fran happy was not good news for me.

"So I went back to my lab and invented this!" she exclaimed as she pulled out a hair dryer.

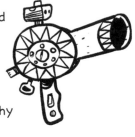

"I think someone else already invented the hair dryer," I told her.

"I know that!" she shouted. "I'm a lot smarter than you, after all! Which is why no one else could have transformed an ordinary hair dryer into an AIR FRYER!"

"Um, I think someone invented that too. Isn't an air fryer a thing you can use to cook French fries and fried chicken?" I asked.

Fran turned red.

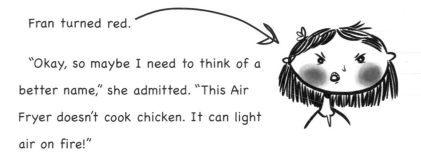

"Okay, so maybe I need to think of a better name," she admitted. "This Air Fryer doesn't cook chicken. It can light air on fire!"

And then she pointed it at me.

"And seeing as you are surrounded by air, that's not good for you." Fran laughed. "It's funny, really – using what used to be a hair dryer to get you out of my hair. Forever!"

I didn't think that was funny at all. I actually found it pretty terrifying. I was so scared, the only parts of me I could get to move were my eyelids. I slammed them shut so I wouldn't have to see what was about to happen to me. But I could still hear as Fran shouted, "Goodbye, ughmmmgh!!"

Huh. That wasn't exactly what I had expected her last words to me to be.

I risked opening an eye (the green one) and saw
Fran on the ground – with Gloria on top of her. She
had tackled Fran just like she had tackled me!

Renfield's barking must have brought Gloria running.
And just in time! I was safe.

But Gloria wasn't.

"Thank you for saving me the trouble of finding
you. You're the one I'm here for," said Fran as her
hand reached towards the Air Fryer, which had fallen
to the ground.

"Look out, Gloria!" I cried.

Gloria looked confused: "Why? What's she going to
do with a hair dry–"

Before I could do anything else, Fran fired!
Suddenly, the air burst into flames!

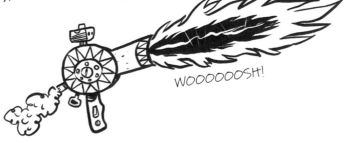

WOOOOOOSH!

Chapter 5

Luckily, Gloria was looking at the Air Fryer when Fran pulled the trigger.

Gloria rolled out of the way just as the air around her caught fire!

The blaze only lasted a second. But that was long enough to melt the bottom of the kiosk advertising tonight's mime show. The heavy kiosk fell over – right on Gloria's legs!

She was hurt. Badly. It didn't look as though she could move her legs.

But that didn't stop her from grabbing the Air Fryer out of Fran's hands and aiming it right back at her!

Fran scrambled to her feet and backed away.

"Don't shoot! I'm going!" she cried. She backed away. "After all, I've got lots more people to visit. Haven't I, JD? You won't be able to get to all of them first!"

As Fran ran off, Gloria tried to get up to chase after her. But Gloria couldn't even get to her feet. She stumbled back to the ground.

That's when I realized I had been standing in the same spot the whole time. I hadn't moved at all!

I raced over to Gloria.

"Are you okay?" I asked. "Are you bleeding?"

"I don't have time to bleed," she replied, as she tried to get to her feet again. "I've got a job to do."

It took all the guts I had to look at her legs.

I don't like blood. So it was lucky for both of us that her legs weren't bleeding. But she couldn't stand.

"This is what happens when a bodyguard doesn't assess risks properly," she said as she looked at the Air Fryer in her hands. "I thought this was just a hair dryer. Now I'm too injured to walk."

"I'm sorry," I told her. "This wouldn't have happened if you hadn't saved me."

"Yes, that was another mistake no bodyguard should make," Gloria nodded sadly. "Leaving her client when danger is present."

"Then why did you do it?" I asked, pretty upset that she had called saving my life a mistake.

"Do you really have to ask, JD?" she said, looking more hurt than when the kiosk had fallen on her legs.

"Well, yeah," I replied. "I mean, you seemed pretty eager to get rid of me. You said I was just a distraction!"

"I did say you were a distraction," said Gloria. "And I meant it. Being a good bodyguard is very important to me, JD. Because it's what my family does. I care about my job because I care about my family."

She looked at me and added, "And you're family, JD."

"When a bodyguard is on duty," she said, "all she's supposed to care about is her client. Having someone like you around that I care about is a distraction."

"Oh," was all I could think to say.

"Now I have to get back to work," she said, all business again. "Get me over to a golf cart."

There was one sitting near by, next to the golf course. I helped Gloria towards the driver's seat.

"The other side," she told me. "You're going to have to drive. My legs can't work the pedals."

I did what she said and got behind the wheel. It was the first time I had driven anything. Which would have been cool, if it weren't for Gloria.

"Which way to the hospital?" I asked as we drove off.

"No hospital," replied Gloria. "Someone still has to protect the Vampire. Drive me back to his house – and fast."

I did what she asked, but I didn't like it. Gloria wasn't bleeding or anything, but her legs probably needed casts or bandages or something.

"Can't the Vampire take care of himself?" I asked her. "I mean, he's the Vampire!"

"He is the Vampire," agreed Gloria as we rode on the golf cart. "But think about it. He's four hundred years old. That's old. And like most really old people, he sleeps all day. Yes, in a coffin instead of on the sofa. But still. He can't even go outside during the day. Twelve hours of every day, he's totally vulnerable unless I'm there to protect him."

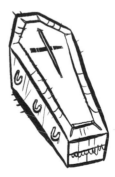

"If he's so allergic to the sun, why is he living here in Miami, Florida?" I asked. "It doesn't get much sunnier than this!"

"I agree," said Gloria. "I told him he'd be much safer in Alaska or Antarctica or somewhere else where the days are short. But he wanted to be here, because he likes to be around older people."

So I had been right!

"You mean because they won't put up a fight when he sucks their blood!" I exclaimed. "And because no one will be surprised if a ninety-year-old dies in the middle of the night!"

"What? No!" said Gloria. "You have some imagination! The Vampire has been a vegetarian for years."

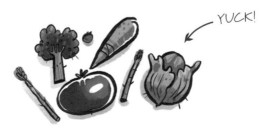

YUCK!

Huh?! So much for my theory. "But if the Vampire doesn't want to bite them, why does he like old people so much?" I asked.

"The Vampire has lived for a long time," Gloria explained as we crossed the last hole of the golf course. "And like most people who have lived a long time, his favourite memories are from when he was younger. The old people who live here are the only ones who know about the things from the 1940s and 1950s that the Vampire likes to remember. Like Frank Sinatra. And black-and-white films."

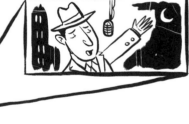

"And mime artists," I added, pointing at a poster of the night's mime show as we drove past it.

"Right," she nodded. "I've never seen a mime show. Have you?"

I shook my head.

"No one under eighty has. That's why the Vampire lives here," said Gloria. "And while I think the sun is an unnecessary risk, there are some things I do like about this place. For one thing, older people tend to eat very bland food. You won't find any garlic around here. That takes away one risk factor. And as a bodyguard, I've got to look out for every risk."

"You make the Vampire sound like a nice person," I said. "So why does he need a bodyguard?"

"Four hundred years is a long time to live. Even the nicest person is going to make mistakes and rub some people the wrong way," she said. "Or in the Vampire's case, one person."

As she said that, Gloria looked around.

"Who?" I asked. "Who are you looking for?"

"Nobody," she replied. "You can't look for someone you can't see."

"What do you mean?" I asked.

But Gloria wasn't listening. We were driving past the Iping Village Community Theatre.

Gloria was looking at a group of men dressed all in black with white painted faces. The mime artists had arrived for their show tonight.

Gloria stared at one of the mime artists. Most were tall and skinny. This one was short and fat.

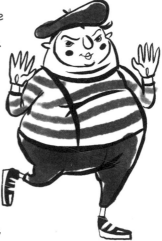

"It's him," whispered Gloria. "He's here!"

Suddenly, the fat mime artist wiped off his face paint. Underneath wasn't a face. In fact, there wasn't anything there at all!

Then he started taking off all his clothes!

There was nothing under them either!

I didn't understand what I was seeing (or not seeing).

Gloria did.

"That's the Vampire's arch-enemy," she told me. "That's the Invisible Man."

Chapter 6

"Drive faster!" cried Gloria. "We've got to get to the Vampire's house before he does!"

I put my foot down as far as it would go, and we raced off.

Well, "raced off" is a bit of an exaggeration. I made the golf cart go as fast as it could, but I probably could have run faster.

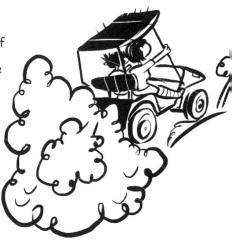

But Gloria couldn't.

"What's happening?" I asked her. "How did that mime artist just disappear?"

"That was no mime artist," said Gloria. "That was the Invisible Man. Remember when I said there was one person the Vampire had rubbed the wrong way? It was the Invisible Man. He must have disguised himself as a mime artist to get through the front gate."

I had never seen anything about the Invisible Man on the internet. But I suppose that made sense. I mean, it's hard to see a lot about someone you can't see.

"He's been trying to get revenge on the Vampire for years," said Gloria. "My family has always stopped him."

"What did the Vampire do to him?" I asked.

Gloria wasn't sure exactly. It had something to do with the Invisible Woman. But whatever it was happened years ago. The Vampire hadn't seen the Invisible Woman in a long time.

"Well, he never actually SAW her," said Gloria. "She is invisible. But, they were going out together behind the Invisible Man's back. Or maybe in front of his back, too. It's hard to tell with invisible people."

"That sounds a bit complicated," I said.

"Not for me," Gloria replied. "When you're a bodyguard, everything is simple. It all comes down to doing whatever it takes to keep your client safe."

We pulled up in front of the Vampire's house. I helped Gloria inside.

In the living room, where the sofa should have been, was a coffin. A huge coffin. It looked like it weighed a tonne (or maybe ten tonnes? How much is a tonne? Anyway, it must have weighed a lot).

"Whoa!" I said. "Is the Vampire..."

"Yes," replied Gloria as she went to the coffin. "The Vampire is safe in there. For now. The coffin can only be opened from the inside. Unless you have this."

She pressed the side of the coffin. A panel popped open. Gloria took out the key that was hidden inside.

"The coffin is indestructible," she explained to me carefully. "The Invisible Man knows he won't be able to get inside and take his revenge unless he has this key."

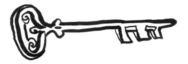

"So why did you just take the key out of its hiding place?" I asked.

"The Invisible Man knows all about the key and the coffin," she replied. "He and the Vampire used to be good friends, remember?"

"Okay, so let's use that key and get the Vampire out of here!" I said.

Gloria looked out through the window. "There's still some time until sunset," she said. "Taking him out of his coffin now would destroy him."

One thing was for sure – we weren't going to move

the Vampire inside the coffin. Whatever made it indestructible also made it incredibly heavy.

OUCH!

"I can't fight the Invisible Man," said Gloria as she took some bandages from the Vampire's bathroom and wrapped up her legs. "And I won't be quick enough to keep the key away from him either."

"Don't panic," I told her. "I'll work something out."

That's what I always said when I found myself in trouble. Sometimes, I said it to pump myself up without totally believing it.

This time, I didn't believe it at all. But Gloria seemed to. She wasn't panicking at all.

"That's correct. You are going to have to work it out, JD," she said. "Because you're the only one who can."

Gloria held up the key.

"According to the Vampire's rules, only a member of my family can protect him," she said.

I started to ask "why", but Gloria held up her card. The one with the "Frequently Annoying Questions".

"I don't have time to explain the Vampire's rules on a normal day," she said. "And this is not a normal day. You're the only one who can do this. But I promised to protect the Vampire. It's what our family has always done."

I was part of that family. I was the only one who could help her. There was just one problem.

"I don't know how to be a bodyguard!" I said.

"All it takes," Gloria told me, "is everything. You have to be willing to do everything you can to make sure nothing happens to the person you're protecting."

She turned and looked me in the eye (the blue one this time). "The only question is," she said, "do you have enough guts?"

I knew the answer immediately. Of course I didn't have the guts!

Chapter 7

I was scared out of my mind. How could Gloria and I be related? Nothing scared her! She had lots more guts than I did!

But then I remembered that the guts she had were inherited from her dad. Which meant they were in me too – because they had been in my dad.

She was family. Now that I'd found her, I didn't want to lose her. And maybe I would, if she tried to protect the Vampire on her own without being able to use her legs.

"Give me the key," I told her. "If you think I can keep it away from the Invisible Man, I'll try my best."

"I never said I thought you could keep it away from him," said Gloria, handing me the key. "I believe the risk is lower with you. I estimate that giving you the key reduces the risk to my client by twenty per cent."

"Whoa – wait!" I exclaimed. "So you're saying I've only got a twenty per cent chance of getting out of here without some crazed person I can't even see grabbing me!?!?"

WHAT????

"No," replied Gloria calmly. "I estimate my odds of evading the Invisible Man with two injured legs are approximately five per cent. Giving you the key increases my client's odds by twenty per cent. In other words, you have a six per cent chance of success."

"Oh," was all I could think to say – before a loud crashing sound made both of us turn our heads towards the door.

BOOM!!!

"The Invisible Man is coming," said Gloria evenly. "Your odds are dropping by the second. I suggest you go. Now."

The door swung open as though it had been kicked in. But no one was there.

Gloria moved to block the door – only to fly off her feet. She hung there, half a metre off the ground.

"Where is the key?" demanded the Invisible Man. "Tell me quickly. I grow tired of holding you aloft."

"Put her down!" I shouted. "I have it!"

"JD, don't," said Gloria, raising her voice for the first time. "This isn't about me!"

It was for me. But I didn't stand around to argue with her. I took off running. And hoped the Invisible Man would follow.

I looked over my shoulder and saw Gloria fall to the ground. She was okay.

But somewhere between me and her was the Invisible Man.

I was glad I had made him leave Gloria without hurting her.

Now I just had to make sure he didn't hurt me!

I raced to a window, pushed it open, and jumped outside.

I hit the ground and started running.

I had two choices: find a way to fight the Invisible Man or find a place to hide.

I suppose that might have been a tough decision for some people.

For me, it was easy. Of course I was going to hide!

I made a loop around the Vampire's house and opened the door to the nearest building.

It was the small community library containing books and board games. Inside, it was dark and empty.

I closed the door quietly behind me, then risked a peek out the window.

I didn't see anything. Nothing at all.

Not even the Invisible Man's face, which was right there staring back at me!

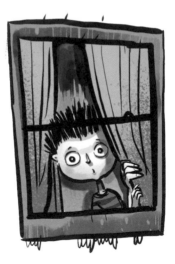

Chapter 8

Of course, I only realized that when – CRASH! – the window smashed in on me.

I could feel a hand grabbing at me. But I couldn't see it. I could only smell the hint of sweat as the Invisible Man struggled to reach me.

I backed away from the broken window.

"I grow weary of this chase," wheezed the Invisible Man, slightly out of breath. "Give me the key."

Suddenly, a sofa floated up and came flying at me. And then a table and a chair.

I dodged the first two. But the chair hit my arm hard.

That's when something else hit me too: the furniture wasn't flying on its own. The Invisible Man was throwing it!

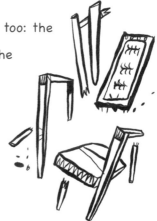

Another chair (a really big one) levitated into the air. But instead of flying at me, it was smashed into pieces.

The message was clear. If the Invisible Man got his hands on me, the same thing would happen to me!

I crept back into the shadows of the darkened library and tried to hide behind a bookshelf.

I was definitely proving how much guts I had.

None.

Then suddenly, I heard a...

CREEEEEEEAK.

It was the bookshelf I was hiding behind. The Invisible Man was right there on the other side, trying to topple it!

"**URRH!**" he groaned as he shoved. He was so close that I could smell his sweat.

The shelf was so overloaded with books, it took him about three seconds of pushing to get it to fall over. Which was just enough time for me to scramble out of the way, as **WHOOMP!** it crashed to the floor.

The Invisible Man had to climb over the fallen shelf, giving me time to run out of the library.

I had to find somewhere else to hide. If he could get that close without me knowing, there's no way I'd escape if he found me again.

Outside, I ran past Renfield, sleeping on the grass.

He lifted his head and let out a loud **WOOOOOF!**

"Shh!" I pleaded. "I need to hide. I know it's not what Gloria would do, but I'm new at trying to be brave and—"

I stopped trying to justify myself to a dog when I realized Renfield wasn't barking at me. But there wasn't anyone else around. Renfield must have been barking at the Invisible Man!

Gloria had said she'd trained Renfield to bark at anyone he hadn't seen before. Well, there was no way Renfield had ever seen the Invisible Man!

But Renfield could smell him. I took off in the opposite direction, silently reminding myself to thank the old dog, if (I mean "when" – stay positive!) I survived all this.

And I really did need to thank him. Not only had Renfield's bark warned me the Invisible Man was close (it certainly would have been great if Renfield could move fast enough to stay with me as I ran) – he had also given me an idea.

Renfield had smelled the Invisible Man. I had, too, when he was close enough to grab me. He was certainly working up quite a sweat chasing after me.

I remembered that when he was dressed as a mime artist, he stood out as being overweight. Which I suppose made sense: if you're invisible, you don't have any motivation to go to the gym to try to look good.

If he was unfit, then the more I could make him run, the sweatier he would get. Perhaps I could get him so sweaty, I could smell his BO coming. I could use my nose instead of my eyes!

I wasn't sure that was a great plan.

In fact, I hoped it really stank!

Chapter 9

I ran for a long time.

That's really all there is to say.

I ran and thought about what the Invisible Man had done to that chair – and hoped he didn't get the chance to do that to me.

***

I must have run for hours. I ran past the theatre, all over the golf course and around the houses. I don't know how many laps I made of Iping Village.

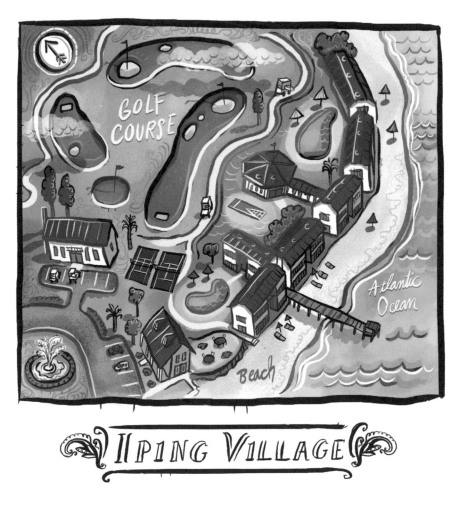

IIPING VILLAGE

In fact, I lost track of time. It was actually pretty boring. Or would have been if I wasn't completely scared out of my mind.

Of course, it would have been easier if I could have just run out of Iping Village and gone somewhere (anywhere) else.

But one whole side of the community ended at the beach. I suppose I could have tried to swim for it. But I was staying ahead of the Invisible Man by running. I didn't know if he'd be faster than me in the water.

The rest of Iping Village was surrounded by a huge fence. There was only one gate. I ran past it a few times, but the security guard had it closed. I didn't have time to stop and explain why he should open it for me, because the Invisible Man was right behind me.

PEWW! I knew that because my plan was working. I could smell his BO a mile away.

Okay, maybe not a mile. But far enough that I had time to run in a different direction when I smelled him getting too close.

As long as I could keep this up, I could keep the key away from him.

There were just a couple of problems with doing that. One: it was a bit embarrassing.

None of the old people were outside to see me. I supposed they were all still taking their afternoon naps, just like the Vampire.

The only people outside were the mime artists, who were holding up the clothes the Invisible Man had been disguised in. They seemed totally surprised that one of them had just disappeared and were trying to tell the security guard what had happened.

Well, they weren't exactly trying to tell him. I suppose they took their miming – or whatever you call it – very seriously. They didn't say a word. They just flapped their arms and waved their hands.

I suppose I can't really blame the guard for looking at them as though they were crazy. I must have looked even crazier to him every time I ran past him as I made my loop of Iping Village. I was running for my life, but he couldn't tell anyone was chasing me.

So I'm sure I looked like a crazy person.

I mean, I am literally sure. Because each time I ran past him, the guard yelled, "What are you doing!?! Are you crazy!?"

As I said, I didn't have time to explain that I wasn't crazy (not that he would have believed me) because the Invisible Man was right behind me.

And anyway, I could handle a little embarrassment.

What I couldn't handle was all the running. One of my legs was shorter than the other, and both of my feet were really huge. That made running difficult.

I was getting tired. Really tired. Pretty soon, I'd have to stop.

Which, on the one hand, would be good. At least I'd stop embarrassing myself in front of the guard.

On the other hand, the Invisible Man would catch me, get the key and do who knows what to the Vampire.

Not to mention me.

I ran out of steam as I was passing the security guard for the nineteenth time.

My legs just wouldn't run anymore. I pitched forwards and collapsed.

Right onto the golf cart next to the security guard!

I hopped in and drove off!

"What're you doing?! Are you crazy?" cried the guard again. "That's my cart. Stop!"

The mime artists all stuck out their palms at me, echoing his calls to stop.

But I didn't listen. (Can you "listen" to people who aren't talking? That sounded like a question I should ask the man I couldn't see. Which I would have if he weren't trying to smash me.)

The security guard hopped onto another golf cart and chased after me.

As he pulled up alongside, I finally had the chance to explain to him that I was being chased by the Invisible Man who wanted the key to the Vampire's coffin that had been given to me by my cousin who was related to me through my dad's large intestine.

Even as I said it, I knew it made no sense.

The guard seemed to agree. "You really are crazy!" he said.

And then he flew out of his golf cart and landed on the ground.

"Hey, who did that?" said the guard as he stumbled to his feet.

I already knew the answer – the Invisible Man.

He got behind the wheel of the guard's golf cart and chased after me. Slowly. Very slowly.

I could have got out and run faster than we were driving.

But I was too tired to run.

Luckily, so was the Invisible Man.

I could hear him wheezing in his
cart. He was too busy catching
his breath to say anything as he
chased me across Iping Village.

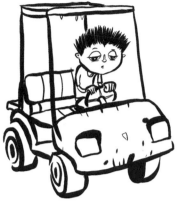

And then suddenly I stopped.

VRRRRRR! My golf cart's wheels kicked up sand. I
had taken a wrong turn and was stuck on the beach!

Having run all over Iping nineteen times, I suppose I
should have known the place better. But it was starting
to get dark and I was too busy being scared out of my
mind to really watch where I was going.

The Invisible Man followed me onto the beach and got
his cart stuck too. But that didn't stop him. I could see
his footprints coming towards me in the sand.

Hey, wait! I could see his footprints in the sand!

I hopped off my cart and ran across the beach.
I had had a bit of rest while driving the golf cart.
Enough to run a little more.

And I knew where to run because I could see the
Invisible Man's footprints under the now-setting sun.
So I knew where he was!

Unfortunately, it wasn't long before the Invisible
Man worked that out. He ran straight into the ocean
(I suppose he had caught his breath too).

The waves were breaking hard. I couldn't tell where
he was in the water.

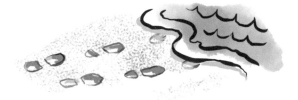

Even worse – the ocean water was like a bath. Now
I couldn't smell him either!

And even even worse – the sun was going down. It
was getting darker.

And even even even worse – well, no. That was as bad as it got. But that was bad enough!

The Invisible Man could have been anywhere. I couldn't smell him. I couldn't see him. It was so dark I couldn't see anything.

Until the air lit up on fire!

"JD! Over here!" said Gloria. She was in another cart at the edge of the sand. She fired another burst from the Air Fryer that lit up the beach.

I saw footprints in the sand. The Invisible Man was coming for me.

And then, just as the flames from the Air Fryer died away, I saw something else.

Next to Gloria, there was someone behind the wheel of the cart. In the dim moonlight, it was too hard for me to see who it was.

Until he rushed right past me, and I saw...

The Vampire!

"No," cried the Invisible Man. "I was going to have my revenge!"

"Yes, you vere," said the Vampire, in whatever type of weird accent the Vampire had. "But dees boy made you vait too long. It ees now night. Too late vor you!"

I really couldn't see what happened next. Between the Vampire's black cape and the Invisible Man being invisible, I couldn't tell what the two were doing in the darkening night.

COOL!

I heard a "Hrnnn!" and then a "Ommph!" and then "**SCRREEECH!**" and then a "**SHOOPH!**" that might have been a hiss of smoke. And then the Vampire and the Invisible Man were gone!

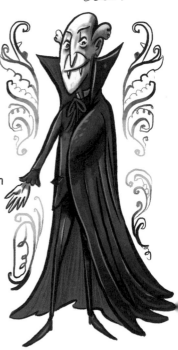

Chapter 10

The next morning, I woke up in the Vampire's house.

No, not in his coffin.

Gloria had invited me to sleep on the sofa. As I slid off it, both my legs ached from all the running I had done the day before. But I couldn't complain about my legs. Gloria had new casts on both of hers.

It would take a little time for them to get better, but that was okay. She had time.

Whatever had happened to the Invisible Man (Gloria wouldn't tell me), he wouldn't be back for a while.

In the meantime, she could get around Iping Village on a golf cart.

I offered to stay and help her, but she said no. I understood. "I suppose I showed yesterday how much help I would be to a bodyguard," I said. "I mean, when things got scary, all I could think to do was run or hide!"

"That's right, JD," she replied. "You did show how much help you could be last night. And all you did was ... save my client!

"What you did last night was the bravest thing I've ever seen," she said. "I told you that you only had a six per cent chance of success, and you agreed to help anyway. Being brave doesn't mean you're never scared. It means that even when things are scary, you still agree to take on the jobs that need to be done."

"You're exactly the kind of person whose help I could use, JD," she said.

"Oh," was all I could think to say. "Thank you."

"You shouldn't be so surprised," said Gloria. "We both got our guts from my father. He was the bravest man I ever knew.

"But I can't let you stay, JD," she went on. "Because you've got another scary job that needs doing. You've got to warn the rest of your cousins about Fran. Now that I know what she looks like, her risk to me is somewhere between low and minimal. Your other cousins are at a much higher risk, if you don't get to them first."

She handed me a bag. After I had fallen asleep on the sofa, the Vampire had returned. He had taken the key back, but before he got back into his coffin (I suppose he was in there right now!), he had left the bag with Gloria to give to me.

"He wanted to give you a little something to thank you for helping to keep him safe," she said.

The bag may have been little, but it was really something. Inside were a handful of gold coins!

"Whoa," I said. "These look old. Are they from the last century?"

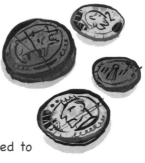

"Try three centuries before that," she told me. "They should be worth enough to get you wherever you need to go to find your next dozen cousins."

Tracking down my first three cousins hadn't been easy. Thinking about what it would take to find the next twelve filled me with a gust of fear. It certainly would have been easier with Gloria's help. But she had a job to do.

So did I. And with the gold coins in one back pocket and my journal in the other, I headed out to do it!

THE END?

GLOSSARY

arch-enemy one's principle or worst foe

kiosk small open-fronted hut usually used to sell newspapers, ice creams or tickets

levitated rise or cause to rise and hover in the air

mime artist performer who expresses himself or herself without words

orphanage place where children who don't have parents live and are looked after

revenge action of hurting or harming someone in return for an injury or wrong caused by them

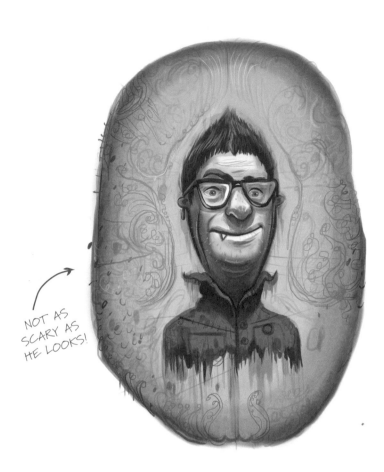

NOT AS SCARY AS HE LOOKS!

Scott Sonneborn has written several books, one script for a circus performance (for Ringling Bros. and Barnum & Bailey), and many TV series. He's been nominated for one Emmy award and spent three very cool years working at DC Comics. He lives in California, USA, with his wife and their two sons.

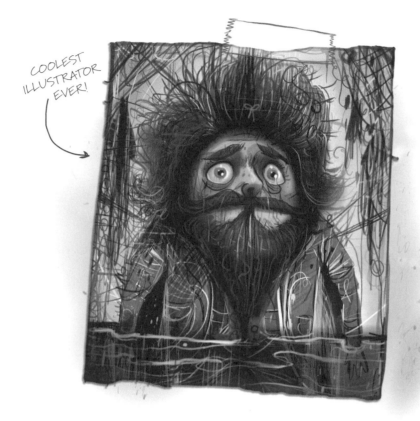

COOLEST ILLUSTRATOR EVER!

Timothy Banks is an award-winning illustrator known for his ability to create magically quirky illustrations for children and adults. He has a Master of Fine Arts degree in Illustration, and he also teaches art students in his spare time. Timothy lives in South Carolina, USA, with his wonderful wife, two beautiful daughters and two crazy pugs.

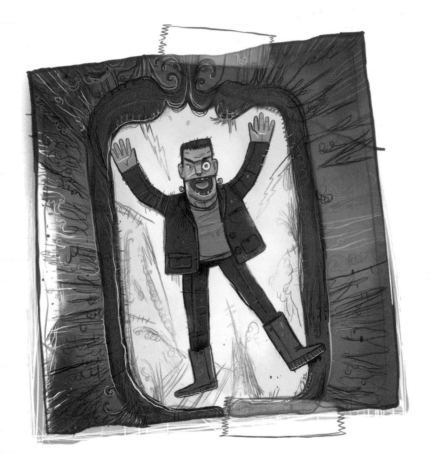